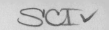

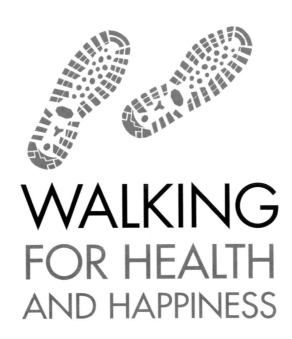

# WALKING

## FOR HEALTH
### AND HAPPINESS

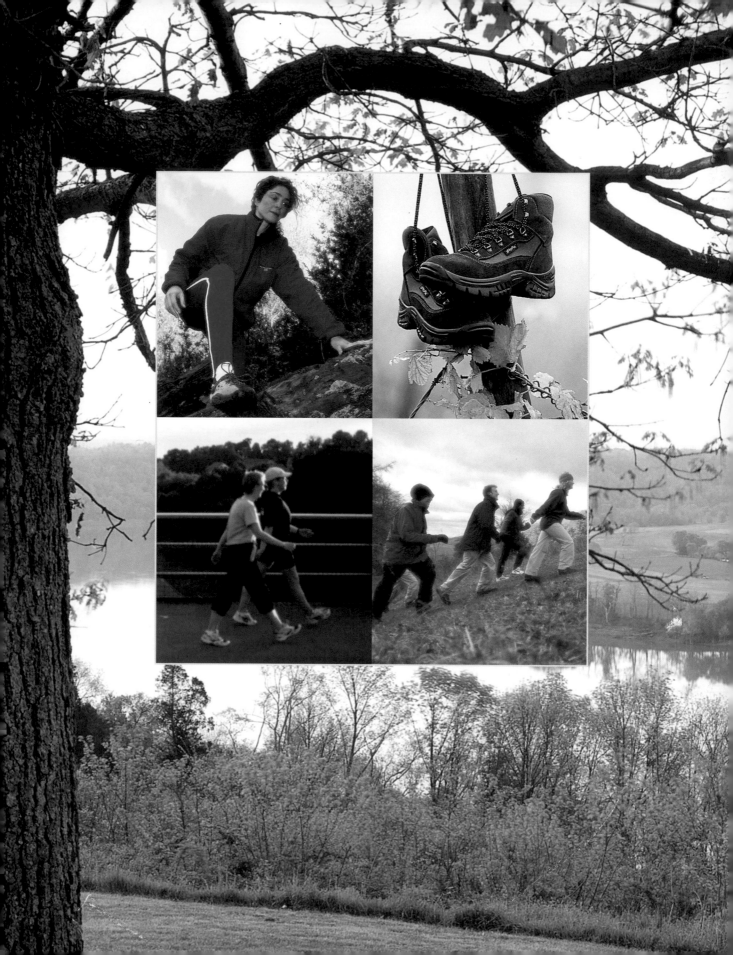

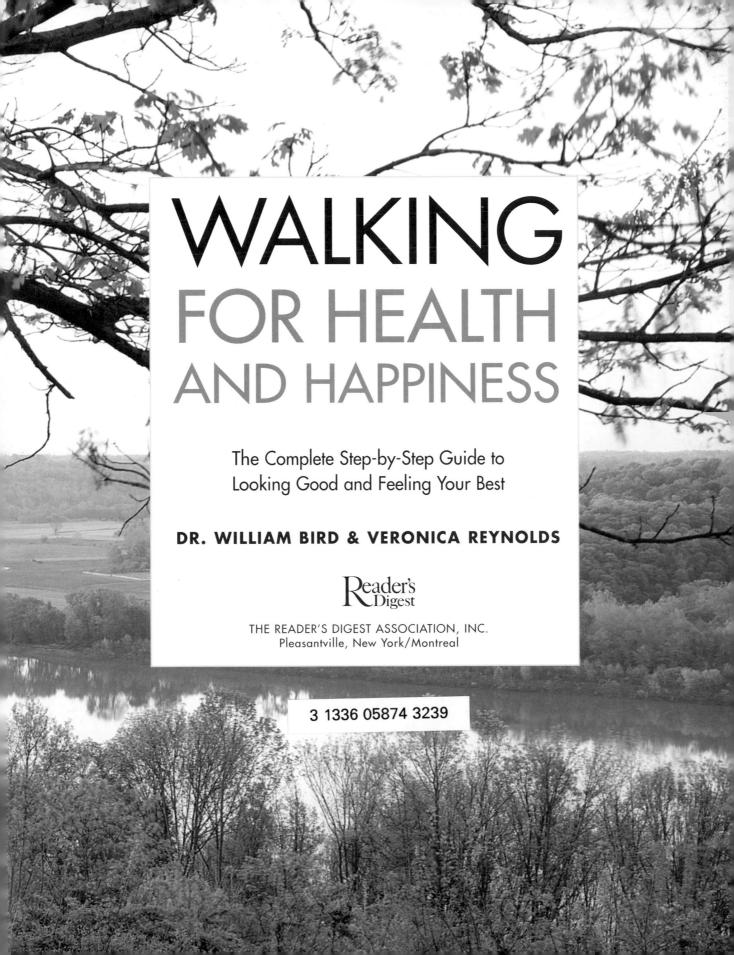

# WALKING
## FOR HEALTH
## AND HAPPINESS

The Complete Step-by-Step Guide to
Looking Good and Feeling Your Best

**DR. WILLIAM BIRD & VERONICA REYNOLDS**

Reader's
Digest

THE READER'S DIGEST ASSOCIATION, INC.
Pleasantville, New York/Montreal

A READER'S DIGEST BOOK

First published in 2002 in the USA by
THE READER'S DIGEST ASSOCIATION, INC.
Reader's Digest Road, Pleasantville, New York 10570-7000, USA

Conceived and produced by
CARROLL & BROWN PUBLISHERS LIMITED
20 Lonsdale Road, Queen's Park, London, NW6 6RD

Managing Editor  Becky Alexander
Project Editor  Kirsten Chapman
Art Editor  Gilda Pacitti
Photography  David Murray, Jules Selmes

Reader's Digest Project Staff
Project Editors  Fred DuBose, Kim Ruderman
Development Editor  Delilah Smittle
Senior Designer  George McKeon
Senior Design Director  Elizabeth Tunnicliffe

Contributing Editors  Barbara Ellis, Barbara Pleasant

Reader's Digest Books
Editorial Director  Christopher Cavanaugh
Executive Editor, Trade Publishing  Dolores York
Director, Trade Publishing  Christopher T. Reggio

Library of Congress Cataloging-in-Publication Data

Bird, William
Walking for health and happiness: the complete step-by-step guide to looking good and feeling your best /
William Bird and Veronica Reynolds.
p. cm.
Includes index
ISBN 0-7621-0364-7
1. Fitness walking. 2. Physical fitness. 3. Health. I.Reynolds, Veronica. II. Title.

RA781.65 .B573 2002
613. 7'176--dc21
2001057890

Visit our online store for more
Readers Digest products and information

Reproduced by P. T. Repro Multi Warna in Indonesia
Printed by Tien Wah Press in Singapore

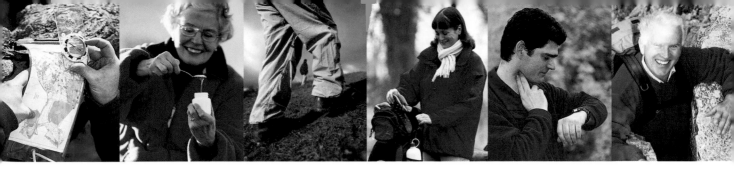

# CONTENTS

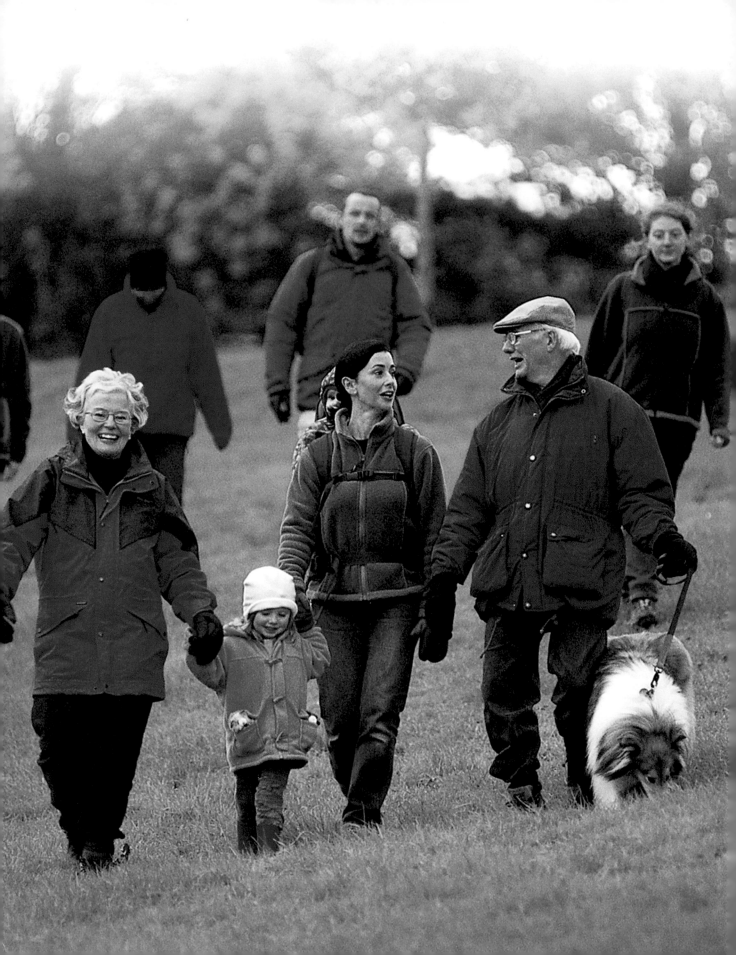

# FOREWORD

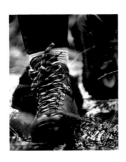

Walking for both health and happiness—are there any better reasons to get up, go out the door, and get moving?

Research has shown that physical inactivity is becoming more prevalent throughout the world. We all know that a sedentary and unfit way of life can be bad for our health, leading to illnesses including heart disease, some cancers, diabetes, obesity, and depression. The high risks associated with inactivity and the number of people who are sedentary combine to make this one of the major public health problems of the 21st century.

So, what can we do about it? Fortunately the remedy is simple—walking for just 30 minutes a day (not necessarily in one session) meets the U.S. surgeon general recommendations for exercise and is feasible for nearly everyone—young and old, healthy and unhealthy, fat and thin, and virtually all groups in the population. Most of us can find time to walk, and it doesn't cost a thing! Dr. William Bird and Veronica Reynolds have written an authoritative, easy-to-use guide that can benefit the tens of millions of people who can improve their lives by investing a mere 30 minutes a day.

I have spent many enjoyable hours over the past 30 years, individually and with family or friends, on my feet and moving through the environment, either in the city or in the country. I have found there is no better way to explore a new city than to go for a walk. Walking allows you to become more in touch with the social and physical environment, providing an appreciation that you cannot get by riding a bus tour or taking a taxi.

This book—packed with scientifically accurate information, helpful tips, good advice, sound behavioral interventions, and other resources—provides the motivation, the knowledge, and the specific how-tos to make physical activity an easy part of everyone's daily lives. *Walking for Health and Happiness* offers not only an enjoyable read but also the inspiration to change lives.

**Steven N. Blair, P.E.D.**
**Director of Research, The Cooper Institute for Aerobics Research, Dallas, Texas**

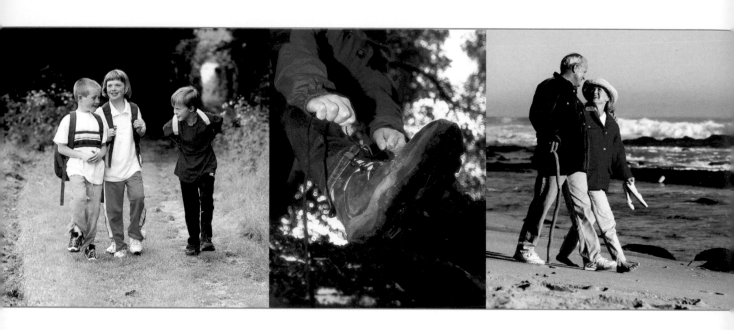

# WHY WALK?

The benefits of walking and the reasons why walking is the perfect exercise for achieving a healthy mind and body at any stage in your life.

1

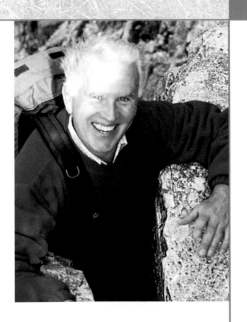

# WALKING IS **FOR EVERYONE**

*Walking is the perfect exercise. Safe, easy and, best of all, free, it benefits the whole body, as well as the mind. This section looks at ways walking can improve your health, even if you suffer from a health condition.*

After four million years of development and improvement, our bodies have been fine-tuned to walk. Evolution has made the ability to walk a priority. Not only have we had to walk for survival—to pick fruit or to reach the river for water—but our bodies also have needed to walk to continue to function normally. In fact, when we stop walking for any length of time, our bodies start to go into decline.

Today, we may no longer need to walk to gather food and water, but our bodies still need regular walking to develop properly. In just 50 years, we have bucked the evolutionary trend our ancestors set into motion. With the proliferation of cars and labor-saving devices, the average person now gets less physical activity in his or her life than at any time in the past. The solution is simple: We need to walk more to stay fit, healthy and happy.

More vigorous exercise, such as jogging or aerobic classes, may achieve fitness results more quickly, but the risk of injury can be high, and such activities are not recommended for those who are unused to a certain level of exercise. Walking, on the other hand, is

### A lifetime of walking
Walking is not just for certain stages of your life. All different age groups, from toddlers to seniors, will enjoy different types of pace and environment.

### Toddlers
The outside world contains lots of distractions that open up a whole new world to explore.

### Children
Variety and interesting terrain will be important. Walking with friends is a time to share confidences.

### Teenagers
Exploration, hiking, and just walking with friends can provide a healthier and more social alternative to other distractions such as watching TV and playing computer games.

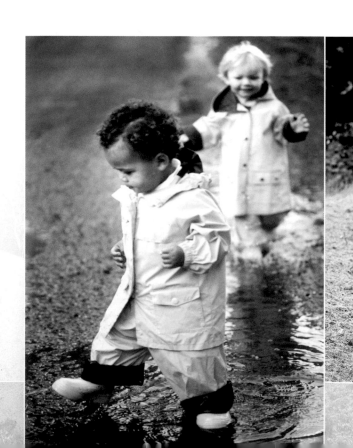

safe, can be enjoyed at every stage of your life and will bring the same health benefits as other more strenuous forms of exercise.

## Is it too late to start?

You're never too old to introduce or increase the amount of walking in your life. From the moment you learn to walk until late in your life, it's a sign of independence and energy. If you want to be fit and full of life in your 80s, you need to include exercise in your life. Keeping active in old age will maintain your quality and enjoyment of life. Bear in mind, however, that although walking brings long-term benefits, you have to exercise regularly to continue to reap them.

## Am I too unfit to start?

Many of the health benefits of walking covered in this chapter—including those for your heart—do not require a huge increase in your level of fitness. It's your increased level of activity that really counts. Even if you haven't exercised for years and have trouble walking up short flights of stairs, professionals recommend walking as the first activity to get yourself back on the road to fitness. Since our bodies are used to walking, the injury rate from walking is lower than for any other type of physical activity. If you know you're very unfit, ease yourself into regular walking with the Beginner's Program on page 150.

Your decision to take up walking is probably not made in a vacuum, but is part of an overall goal to introduce physical activity into your everyday life. If you want to maximize the benefit you get from walking, think about making other health decisions at the same time, such as stopping smoking, adopting a healthier diet and reducing cholesterol, and cutting down on your alcohol intake. Tell your doctor that you've decided to start on a program of regular walking and discuss your overall health plan with him or her.

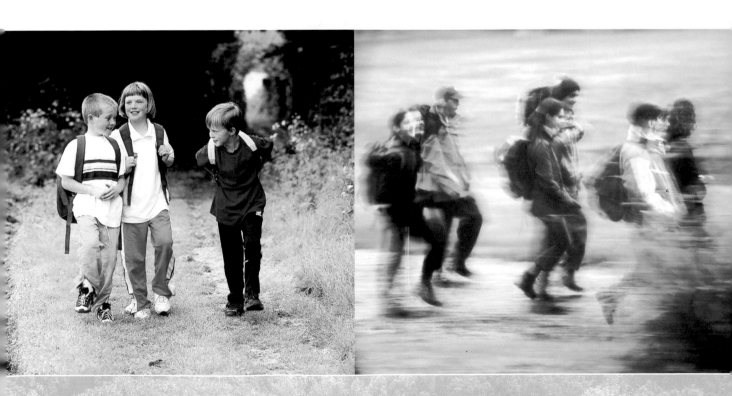

## How much walking do I need to do?

The ideal amount of walking, according to many health organizations and the U.S. surgeon general, is a total of 30 minutes a day for at least five days a week. At first, this may sound like a lot, but this book will show you how to introduce walking into your life in ways that are both achievable and enjoyable.

Your goal should be to take advantage of every single walking opportunity you have, and to walk regularly. If you don't have time for the full 30-minute walk on one particular day, because you have to go to the store, visit a neighbor, then pick up the kids from school, don't worry. This doesn't mean that you have to abandon your walking altogether. Dividing the 30 minutes into three 10-minute sessions will bring just as many health benefits. When you wake up in the morning, or before you go to bed the night before, think about the activities that lie ahead that day. Then rethink them as potential "opportunities for walking." Write a letter you could have sent by email or fax simply because this will force you to walk to the mailbox and back again. Instead of calling in an order for pizza for the kids, walk to the pizza shop, then walk around the block while it's being made.

Many people feel they get enough exercise to remain healthy, but in fact, only 30 percent of us actually do. Make a note of the amount of exercise you got last week. How often did you exercise, take a walk, use the stairs, and so on? It may be surprising to discover how little we exercise during an average week. Continue to make notes as you gradually bring walking into your life. This will help you stay motivated.

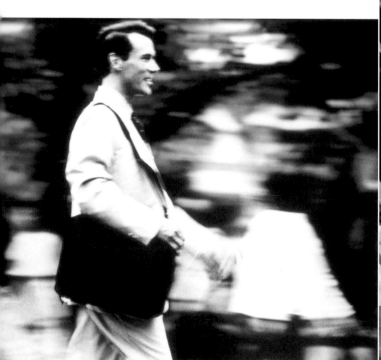

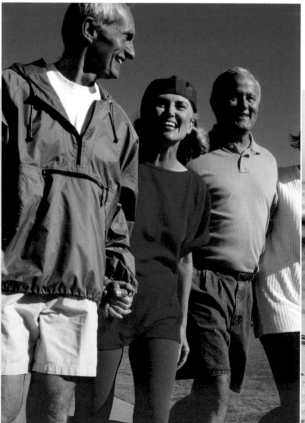

# WALKING *for health and happiness*

▶ Regular walking can produce a more efficient heart, help you lose weight and gain strength, stamina and flexibility—all of which help you live longer and improve your quality of life.

▶ Exercise improves your circulation, which gives your skin a fresher, healthier look.

▶ If you're suffering from stress or anxiety, a brisk walk will help you put problems in perspective.

▶ Walking is an ideal time to meet up with friends, family or a group, to chat and share experiences.

▶ Walking can help with many health conditions, such as diabetes, heart problems, osteoporosis, back pain, asthma and bronchitis.

▶ Increasing your levels of activity can help you sleep better at night, which benefits your overall health and well-being.

*"Take a 2-mile walk every morning before breakfast."*

HARRY TRUMAN

*Advice given on his 80th birthday on how to live to be 80.*

## Is all walking equal?

One of the great things about walking is the variety it offers. Outdoor walking, from a stroll in the park to a challenging hike, lets you explore many different types of terrain and brings health benefits from being in the open air. Indoor walking, in malls, on treadmills, or even up and down the stairs or along corridors, provides an all-weather alternative.

All types of walking are beneficial to your health. Try out as many different types as you can, find out which ones you like best and always remember that variety is the key.

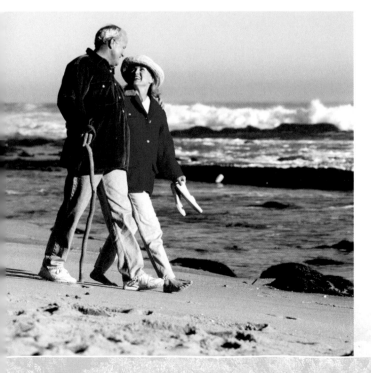

### Adults

With so many responsibilities, the task is to find opportunities in your busy day. Walk to work or take a walk at lunchtime. Abandon the car for short trips like walking to the store or picking up the kids from school.

### 50+

When the kids have left home, walking can help you explore your new-found freedom. Join an organized group to widen your social circle and make new friends.

### Retirement

Take advantage of your extra free time by going on vacations where you can walk in scenic places. Or create a daily routine that incorporates a walk in a safe environment.

# THE **PHYSICAL BENEFITS**

*Walking can improve your whole body considerably—
helping you lose weight, strengthening your heart,
muscles and bones, making you more flexible and
boosting your immune system to fight off disease.*

Health professionals outline three main types of fitness—cardiovascular fitness, musculoskeletal strength and flexibility—and these can all be helped by walking (see opposite). Walking also affects many other aspects of health: maintaining your body weight, boosting immunity, improving your breathing, aiding deep and restful sleep and helping your metabolic fitness—which refers to your body chemistry, such as cholesterol and insulin levels.

## Improving your heart health

Regular walking has many positive effects on the heart and circulation. For example, it strengthens and improves the efficiency of the heart and makes blood flow faster and freer around the body. But the most dramatic fact is that regular walking cuts your risk of a heart attack in half. Inactivity is a high-risk occupation. It has the same effect on your heart as smoking 20 cigarettes a day, having high blood pressure or a high cholesterol level. According to recent research from the National Heart Forum, London, if we all walked the recommended minimum of 30 minutes, five days a

week, 37 percent of heart attacks could be prevented. In addition to this, walking helps by:

- Lowering blood pressure and cholesterol levels, even if these are already high
- Reducing the stickiness of the blood, which helps prevent clots and improves your circulation
- Promoting weight loss, which reduces the work-load on the heart

Walking is a low-impact, weight-bearing exercise and compares favorably with other cardiovascular fitness activities. If you've been advised by your physician to get more exercise for heart-health reasons or you're recovering from heart problems, walking is the perfect exercise for you (see the Walking for a Healthy Heart program on page 156).

## Improving flexibility

With every step you take on your walk, you'll be stretching the muscles in your body and increasing your flexibility and range of movement. Walking works the muscles of the legs and feet the hardest, but if you swing your arms as you walk, you'll be improving the flexibility of your upper body, too. Different types of walking benefit particular muscles more—for example, uphill walking is great for your calf muscles.

Stretching exercises are an essential part of your walking program—bear in mind that they must be performed regularly to increase your flexibility.

### PREVENTING STROKE

Women who engage in moderate exercise, including walking, can reduce their risk of having a stroke, according to a recent study by Harvard University. The study monitored 72,488 female nurses ages 40 to 65 over a period of 15 years. The results showed that for every hour spent in moderate to vigorous physical activity each week, which includes brisk walking, stroke risk was cut by roughly 10 percent—even for those women who had previously been inactive.

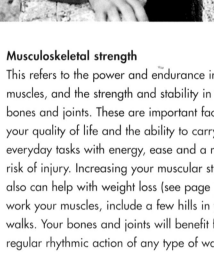

### Cardiovascular fitness

This refers to the efficiency of your heart and circulatory system at taking in oxygen and transporting it around your body and to your muscles. Because it involves these life-sustaining systems, it's perhaps the most important type of fitness to work on. Moderate activities that are sustained for a period of 20 minutes or more and repeated regularly are recommended for improving your cardiovascular fitness. Walking is just such an activity. For the best results you need to walk fast, but without overexertion.

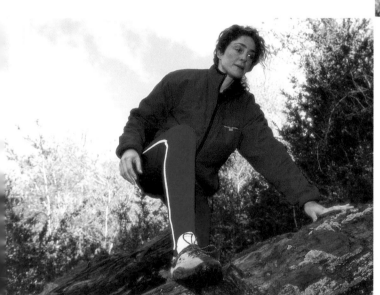

### Musculoskeletal strength

This refers to the power and endurance in your muscles, and the strength and stability in your bones and joints. These are important factors for your quality of life and the ability to carry out everyday tasks with energy, ease and a reduced risk of injury. Increasing your muscular strength also can help with weight loss (see page 16). To work your muscles, include a few hills in your walks. Your bones and joints will benefit from the regular rhythmic action of any type of walking.

### Flexibility

Flexibility means having a full range of movement in your joints and muscles. The more flexible you are, the better you can stretch to reach a book on a high shelf, bend to tie your shoelaces or twist to look over your shoulder. Flexibility is achieved by taking your joints through their range of motion—the sort that you get with each step of a walk—and regular stretching—such as when you do the cool-down exercises on pages 40 to 43.

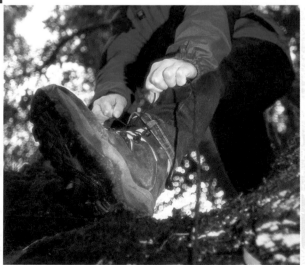

## Helping muscles and bones

If we want to maintain our independence into later life, we should work at building our musculoskeletal strength. However, those people who already suffer from pain and illness in these areas need not give up exercise, as it can actually bring pain relief and health improvements. Walking is particularly beneficial as it is gentle and low-risk, yet effective.

### Walking to help arthritis

Walking is the ideal activity to help reduce the pain and stiffness of arthritis. Osteoarthritis occurs when cartilage around the joint wears away. This means that the joint moves around more and can become very painful. Rheumatoid arthritis is a more serious condition, and if you suffer from this type of arthritis, check with your doctor before taking up walking. With regular walking, the muscles around the joint become stronger and stabilize it, therefore reducing the movement of the joint and halting the progression of the osteoarthritis.

If you have arthritis in your hips or knees you may find that walking becomes difficult, and this can lead to weight gain and additional problems with the arthritis. But you shouldn't be discouraged. Start slowly and you will be surprised how your distances will gradually increase as your joints become more flexible.

### Walking to help bone strength

More than 25 million people in the United States are afflicted with osteoporosis—a condition that can lead to painful fractures of the spine and hips. Regular walking, particularly if it includes some hills, can improve flexibility, balance and muscle strength, all of which help reduce fractures by 30 to 40 percent. Greater flexibility and muscle strength in your back reduces the chance of fractures of the vertebrae, improves posture and lowers the risk of curvature of the spine (kyphosis).

## BEATING BREAST CANCER

In a 2001 study, published in the journal, *Epidemiology*, almost 2,500 women, half of whom had developed breast cancer and half of whom hadn't, were questioned about their level of activity. Those who took up exercise after menopause had a 30 percent reduced risk of developing breast cancer, while those who had exercised regularly throughout their lives had a 42 percent reduced risk.

### Walking to help back pain

Back-pain sufferers are sometimes reluctant to take up walking, thinking that it's going to make the problem worse. In fact, the opposite is true. Walking helps to improve posture and reduce back pain. It increases the strength of the back muscles without putting undue strain on them. As Chapter 2 will show, it's best if you walk with your body held upright and tall, maintaining this position for the length of your walk. Walking tall also strengthens the stomach muscles, which help support the back.

## Walking off a few pounds

Being overweight can affect your health and your confidence, but walking can help you to lose weight—and keep it off. Walking a few times a week helps control weight, but for maximum benefit, aim to walk 30 minutes a day at least five days a week. This might sound like a lot, but you can divide it into short walks taken throughout the day and still reap the benefit. If you keep at this level and include a few hills, you might be able to lose up to 4 lbs (1.8 kg) a month, and that's without dieting. Of course, being overweight has health problems associated with it, such as increased risk of heart disease, diabetes and joint problems, so weight loss from walking will improve your health in these areas, too.

Physical activity helps you lose weight by burning calories. It also improves your basal metabolic rate (see page 158) and your body's ability to extract energy from fat cells. If you have a normally sedentary lifestyle and your body has to cope with a sudden burst of activity, it will take energy from its emergency energy stores in your blood sugar. This energy needs to be replaced quickly, which may be why after physical exertion you crave high-fat foods like candy, potato chips and cookies. With regular walking, enzymes in the body that can extract energy from fat cells become more active and your emergency supplies are left untouched, reducing the urge to snack. This depletion of fat cells, together with an improved diet, leads to weight loss.

The ideal healthy lifestyle is to combine a sensible diet with regular physical activity. If you remain overweight but are physically active, you're still more healthy than someone who is of normal weight but not active. Therefore, walking helps weight control by:
- Reducing the health problems of being overweight
- Lowering weight gradually so it can be kept off
- Promoting the effects of a good diet
- Helping stop the urge to snack
- Toning your muscles so your body looks slimmer

## Walking to fight disease

The more regular walking you do, the less chance you have of catching a cold or picking up an infection. This is because moderate levels of exercise have been shown to enhance the immune system, helping it fight off illness and reduce the incidence of certain cancers. Many doctors also advocate exercise to aid recovery from an illness or surgery. This is because any activity increases your blood flow and raises oxygen levels in the areas that are recovering. Oxygen stimulates the immune system to help repair damaged tissue. Unfortunately, however, the benefits are short-lived. You need to walk every day to continue to boost your immune system.

One of the most remarkable benefits of regular walking, according to a 1996 report by the U.S. surgeon general, is that it halves your risk of developing colon cancer. Colon cancer is the second highest cause of cancer deaths in the United States and Canada. Regular walking also can reduce the risk of developing breast cancer, which claims the lives of 46,000 Americans and 5,500 Canadians each year. A recent study, in the *Archives of Internal Medicine*, showed that 7 hours of walking a week at a brisk pace of 3 to 4 mph (5 to 6.5 km/h) was associated with a 20 percent reduction in the incidence of breast cancer.

Regular walking, by decreasing the amount of fat around your belly, can help lower your insulin levels considerably, therefore lowering your risk of cancer. Maintaining insulin levels is a particular benefit, too, to those who suffer from diabetes (see pages 106 to 107).

## BOOSTING IMMUNITY explained

We have several lines of defense in our highly complex immune systems. The skin, mucous membranes and various proteins, chemicals and cells all enable our bodies to repel, recognize and destroy foreign bodies and abnormal cells. The natural killer (NK) cell is just one of these defenses and it has a particular relationship with exercise. NK cells constantly monitor the areas germs can enter, such as the digestive tract, nose and lungs. Unlike other white blood cells, the NK cells immediately destroy any cell they do not recognize, assuming it's an enemy. In this way, they protect against a large number of infectious organisms. They are also known for their ability to kill cancer cells. Exercise has been proven to boost immunity by increasing the activity of NK cells.

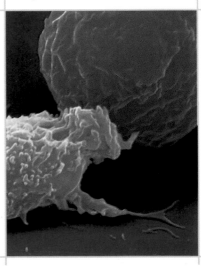

# THE **EMOTIONAL BENEFITS**

*The benefits of regular walking go far beyond the benefits of physical fitness alone. Finding time to get outside and go for a walk can boost your self-esteem and generally make you feel more in control of your life.*

Walking distracts us from the worries of daily life, giving our minds a much needed rest. The more walking the better, but even after a 5-minute walk the body will release endorphins, its natural antidepressant. Walking is also one way of achieving a personal goal, which can help build confidence. Walking can help relieve the physical symptoms of stress and depression, such as tense shoulders and headaches. The social benefits and sheer pleasure of being outside lift the spirits; many people find a walk the ideal time in which to explore their spiritual sides.

### Walking away from depression

With about 1 in 20 young people and 1 in 7 of the elderly suffering from depression, we should all try to protect ourselves from this debilitating condition. It can damage our relationships, careers and physical health. Anxiety, another common condition, is defined as excessive worry and tension. At least 1 person in 20 is said to suffer from anxiety.

Recent research has shown that exercise can be an extremely effective treatment for the symptoms of depression, particularly when combined with

> *"The true charm of pedestrianism does not lie in the walking, or in the scenery, but in the talking."*
> **MARK TWAIN**

conventional treatments. This finding has been ascribed to the release of endorphins. These are proteins released from the brain, which act on the nervous system to reduce pain and elevate mood. Walking is an activity that releases large quantities of endorphins, and these provide you with an instant, natural feel-good factor. Walking briskly for half an hour, five days a week has been shown to be the ideal amount of exercise for those at risk of depression or anxiety. Benefits become evident after four weeks, and maintaining this level of activity helps prevent symptoms from recurring. The walking program on pages 168 has been specifically designed to help with both these conditions.

### Walking away from stress

We are all familiar with the symptoms of stress: tension, anxiety, irritability and sleeplessness. When concerns and worries start interfering with your daily life, you feel "stressed." The muscles around your temples or in the back of the neck tighten. A headache can result. Walking can offer excellent relief from stress; if you go to green, open spaces or a wooded area, away from traffic and noise, you can feel your stress levels decrease within a few minutes. In the long term, regular walking can also help you cope with difficult situations at home or work.

### Social benefits

Modern lifestyles have reduced our levels of social interaction, and isolation is now considered by many health organizations to be a risk factor for disease and illness. Walking is an excellent way to get out and improve your social opportunities. Walking with a group is fun and safe and exercising in the company of others will encourage you to keep walking. Even walking on your own allows you to tune into community life and increases your chance of meeting a new neighbor.

## Walking to lift the spirits

Every walk is a new experience that can have a positive influence on our well-being. Take the same route every day and there will always be something new to see—whether it be a person you meet, the changing flora, or the movement of clouds. It can be just as uplifting to walk in a bustling, energetic city, watching people move through their daily lives.

Human beings have an instinctive desire to feel a part of the natural world; medical professionals have termed this "biophilia" and have started to recognize

that being outdoors has a positive effect on the quality of people's lives. In one study, Professor Roger Ulrich, an environmental psychologist at Texas A&M University, found that hospital patients who had views of trees from their beds recovered more quickly than those who could see only a wall.

Many people find also that their walking time is an opportunity for them to get in touch with their spiritual side. Solitary walking, ideally in a beautiful and tranquil setting, can be a time for meditation and prayer, away from the pressures of daily life. And what better place to do this than the great outdoors?

**Humans are social creatures**
*Walking in groups is an ideal way to keep in touch with neighbors and other members of your community.*

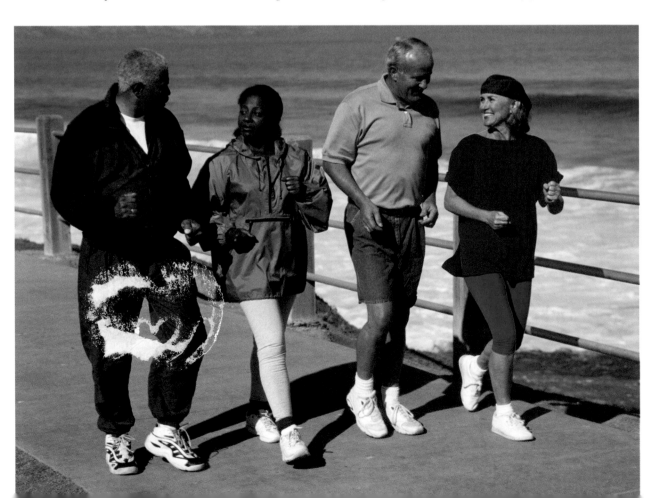

# **MOTIVATION** TROUBLESHOOTER

*If you've bought this book, then you've already taken the first step toward walking more. But is there anything stopping you from getting started? If any of these excuses sound familiar, here are a few solutions.*

**With all the other things going on in my life, how am I going to find 30 minutes a day to go walking?**

It's true, a small adjustment may be needed, but once you begin to feel the benefits, you'll realize that this is a small sacrifice to make. There may be a short walk you can take at lunch or a regular weekend walk, or try breaking up your walking into two or three shorter periods. The clock is ticking, and for each day you're not active your body suffers. The question really is, "can I afford not to spend 30 minutes a day walking?"

**I have young children. How can I go out walking?**

Taking children on a walk can be challenging, but if you motivate them properly the benefits to both their health and yours will be considerable. Carrying very young children on your back or pushing them in a stroller will increase your own strength and stamina.

**I get out of breath going on a short walk. Am I too unfit to start a program?**

If you're simply unfit then walking is the easiest way to get back in shape. If you're getting unduly out of breath, feeling dizzy or experiencing chest pain when walking, then see your physician. You may just need to go at a slower pace until you build up your fitness.

**At the end of the day, I'm too tired to do any exercise. Where am I going to find the energy?**

One of the reasons you may be feeling sluggish is because you're not getting enough exercise. People who have started walking say time and again that they have gained more energy, stamina and a greater feeling of well-being as a result of the increased activity.

**I suffer from a health condition. Is this going to stop me from walking?**

There are very few health problems that prevent you from walking. These are covered on pages 96 to 97. In fact, the majority of physical conditions will be improved by regular walks.

**Doesn't walking get repetitive?**

Once you've been walking for a few weeks, you may feel that you could be doing something more or different. The trick is to challenge yourself. Increase the intensity of your walks (see pages 44 to 53), change the type of walk, explore new locations or join a group to meet new people (see Chapter 3).

**I don't like walking in the cold and rain or when it's too hot. Where can I walk?**

Don't let the weather stop you. If you put on your waterproof clothing and go out for a walk in the rain you might actually find it invigorating. Alternatively, go to the gym and walk on a treadmill (see page 46), or visit your local mall for some climate-controlled walking (see page 70).

**I live in the city. Where can I find an enjoyable walk?**

Cities can be great places to explore. There may be the perfect spot just around the corner, but you won't discover it until you start walking. If there really is nowhere local, it's worth making a short ride to reach a suitable area that you'll really enjoy once you're there.

**I feel nervous about walking on my own, especially at night. What can I do?**

Make time for your walk during your lunch break and walk in populated places, or consider joining a group (see pages 60 to 63). Alternatively, start walking with a friend. That way you'll be able to encourage one another to keep up the exercise.

**I'm not really a fitness fanatic. Don't you need a lot of gear to do this sort of thing?**

That's the beauty of walking. You're bound to have something suitable to wear at home, or be able to get hold of a reasonably priced pair of shoes (see page 123), and once you've mastered the basic technique (see page 26), there's nothing stopping you.

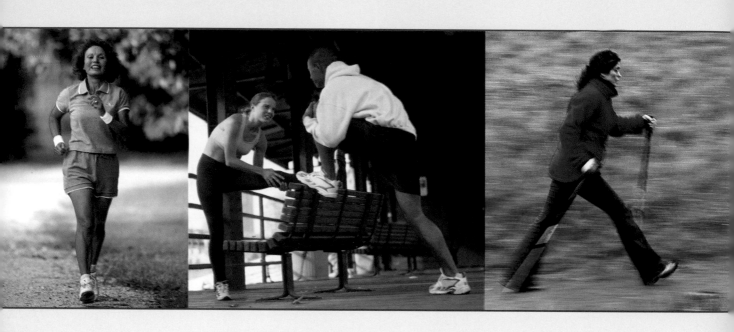

# WALKING
# TECHNIQUES

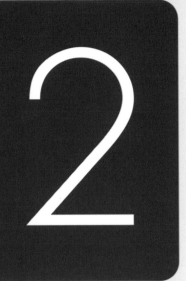

## 2

*The posture, foot placement, breathing, warm-ups and cool-downs that will help you to walk safely and effectively and get the best out of your exercise.*

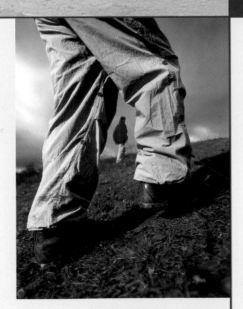

# THE **BASIC TECHNIQUE**

*Walking is an activity that should come naturally and be uncomplicated. Yet many of us still do it badly. This section shows how good posture and correct breathing will help you get the most from your walking.*

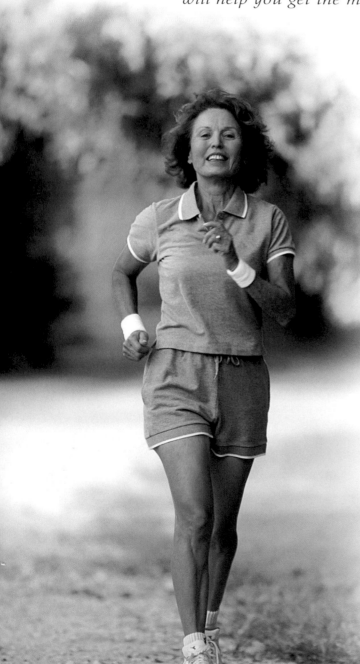

It's perhaps a reflection of how little we use walking as a mode of transportation that we have become so bad at it. If you observe people in Africa or Asia as they walk, you'll see that they appear to glide along, regardless of the fact that they may well be carrying loads of up to 90 lbs (41 kg) on their heads. In contrast, observe people in any Western city: Some of them will be walking with ease, but many will look quite uncomfortable. Often this is a result of carrying too much weight around the waist, but usually it's just bad posture. We seem to have largely ignored our mothers' instructions to "stand up straight," and now slump along, hands in our pockets, dragging our feet, heads down and shoulders hunched. There is no doubt also that our choices of footwear and clothing often severely restrict our abilities to walk effectively, so walking becomes hard work. On the other hand, the good news is that "proper" and efficient walking is something that nearly everyone can learn.

## Why good technique is important

Planes, trains and automobiles all have moving parts. They are rigorously tested by manufacturers to make sure these parts work smoothly and efficiently for their

### Walk tall, stay strong

*As you walk, imagine a string in the top of your head that's pulled toward the sky. This will keep your back straight and your chest open for optimal breathing.*

projected lifetime. On a smaller scale, a prototype kitchen drawer, for example, will be opened and shut hundreds of times during its production, to test that its construction and operation are flawless. One slight off angle can, over time, lead to a serious malfunction.

The human body is not so different. If we use it incorrectly, then—perhaps not immediately, but with repeated use—it becomes stiff or injured. So it's important to adopt a near-perfect walking technique. Good posture and foot placement prevent injury and discomfort, so spend the first few weeks of your program perfecting your technique. This may mean walking more slowly than you would normally until you get the hang of it. But you'll know that when you rebuild your speed, you're doing so safely.

## Building speed

If you think there's little to walking except putting one foot in front of the other, you may be surprised at how much technique can affect your walking. Once you've perfected your posture and breathing, your walking can improve dramatically, allowing you to walk farther and faster, and get much more out of exercise.

If you join a group of walkers, you may be astonished initially by the pace that some of the regular walkers achieve. It's not, however, their level of fitness alone that propels them, it's their practice of good walking technique. It's easy to underestimate what good posture and technique can do for your walking speed, and how quickly you can improve once you've mastered the basics.

## Progress when ready

To develop your fitness from walking, you will, at some point, need to start walking faster, for longer periods or with more intensity (see page 44). Once you are used to the basic walking technique, a brisk pace should be your goal; the benefits covered in Chapter 1 will be achieved only if you continually push your body beyond its usual capacity. Although there's much enjoyment achieved from strolling, you'll soon find that brisk walking is exhilarating and rewarding. This chapter introduces you to simple ways you can get more from your walks. To gauge your current level of fitness and learn how to devise your own walking program, see page 148.

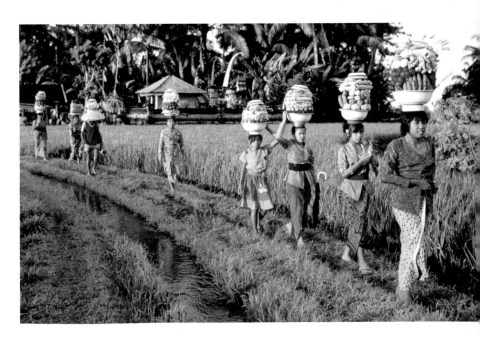

**A natural walk**
*People who walk because it's their major mode of transportation do so gracefully and seemingly effortlessly.*

## The form for fitness

Many different parts of the body, all operating together, are used when you're walking, so you need to consider your whole body posture to perfect your technique. A good way to remember it all is to work systematically from your feet up to your head. Using the following basic walking techniques should not cause you pain or discomfort, but may feel different from the way that you normally walk. Good posture will, in fact, help protect you from strains and injuries. When you're walking hills or doing a walk-run you'll need different postures (see pages 48 and 52).

### Your feet

The foot, one of the most complex structures in the human body, has 26 bones, 33 joints, 19 muscles and 107 ligaments. It has to adjust to various forces and to many different terrains. As you move your foot through the gait cycle (see box, below), the foot changes from a flexible structure, which absorbs impact, to a rigid structure, which transfers force, and then back again to a flexible structure, ready for the next step. The arches play a crucial part in this. Consisting of ligaments, reinforced by tendons, they act like two curved springs, side by side. Together with the heel and calf, the arches provide the "spring in your step."

### Your legs

The muscles in your legs and knees should be relaxed and loose as you walk. Don't lock your knees during either the heel strike or the push-off (see box, below) and keep them a little bit apart. A stiff straight leg will put undue pressure on your knee joints.

### Your torso

Keep your torso straight and pull your belly in. When you're breathing deeply, however, you will have to allow a little room for movement (see page 30). Tuck

## FOOTWORK

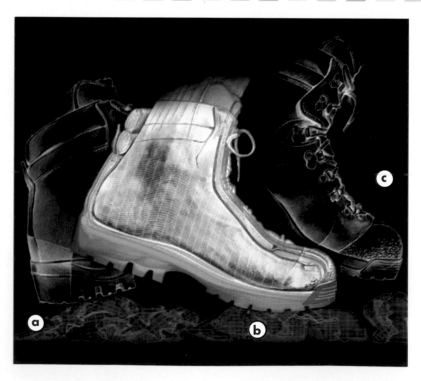

As you take a step **a,** your heel hits the ground first. Your knee unlocks and your foot relaxes, to absorb impact and conform to the terrain. This is the "heel strike." Your weight should roll down the outside of your sole and across the ball of your foot **b** toward your big toe. As your other leg swings, the knee of your supporting leg bends slightly and the calf contracts so your ankle can bend forward. This causes your heel to lift so you can continue pushing off from the ball of your foot to your big toe **c.** Avoid lifting your foot until the big toe has made contact.

your pelvis under slightly so your butt does not stick out. This will keep your lower back strong and prevent strains. When people are told to "straighten up," they tend to adopt a rigid posture, shoulder blades pulled back and chests forced out. Instead of "straight," think "tall." Lengthen your back and keep your chest open.

## Your arms and shoulders

A walk is a time for relaxation—hunched shoulders may be a sign of stress. Try to keep shoulders loose and down, and free of tension. Let your arms swing naturally in opposition to your legs, with elbows bent and hands loosely cupped, as though you are holding a potato chip (see box, above). Your arms should propel you almost as much as your legs.

## Your head and neck

Keep your head comfortably balanced and prevent excessive neck movement. Don't lean your head to the left or right. Try not to look at your feet all the time as this will strain your neck. You can look down occasionally but mostly keep the eyes level.

## ARM CONTROL

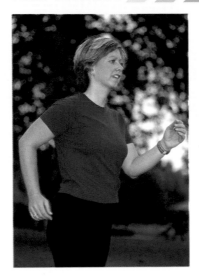

Bend your arms at 90 degrees at the elbows and keep your arms low when coming forward. They should rise no higher than chest level. Swing your arms close to your body, with your hand brushing your hip, and make sure that you're moving your arms forward and backward, rather than side to side. Check the shape of your hands—they should be loosely cupped in a partially closed curl, not clenched.

**Keep a level head**
*The most comfortable position for your head and neck will be achieved if you keep your chin parallel to the ground and look at a point about 15 ft (4.5 m) in front of you.*

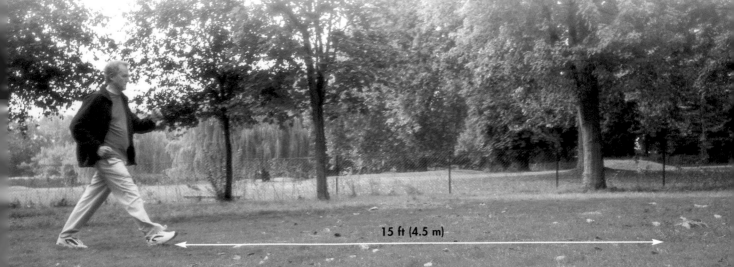

15 ft (4.5 m)

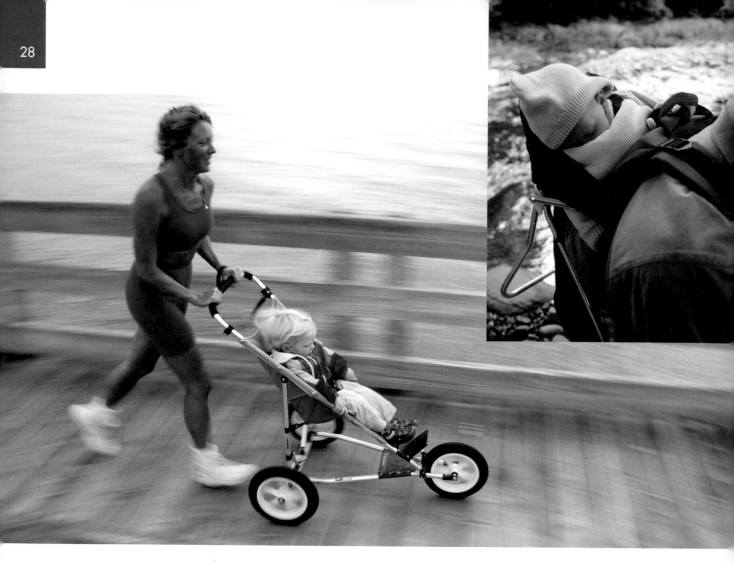

## Dealing with posture problems

Even small imbalances in your posture can lead to strain and possible injury. Carrying a water bottle in one hand or even a personal stereo can throw the body out of line. Whenever possible, use a belt, fanny pack or day pack to carry items you need on your walk.

### Walking with a backpack

Research has shown that carrying a load high on the back requires less energy, so if you're taking a backpack or day pack, make sure that you wear the shoulder straps and hip belt (if you have one) reasonably tight and evenly adjusted, so that the pack is level, doesn't wobble from side to side, and sits fairly high on your back. Make sure you know how to pack items so that the weight is evenly distributed. The best way to spread the load in a large backpack is discussed on page 133.

### Walking with a baby

One of the best exercises for a new mom is walking, but now there are two of you to think about. Jogging strollers are available widely; they have three wheels and maneuver more easily on rougher surfaces, so you'll be able to take your child on all your usual walking routes.

Pushing a stroller, however, will compromise your technique. You'll not be able to swing your arms properly, and good posture in your back is harder to maintain. To minimize the strain on your lower back, use your whole body to push the weight of the stroller. Keep your arms bent just at about waist height, and walk tall, without sticking your butt out.

An alternative is to use a backpack-style child carrier. Your arms will be free to move, and this will help with your balance and propulsion. You'll also have

## Taking baby along

*While toddlers will enjoy being pushed in a three-wheel jogging stroller, younger babies can be carried on your back and infants in a front-facing carrier.*

## Share the fun

*Having your dog along can make a walk more varied—you don't know what you two might discover.*

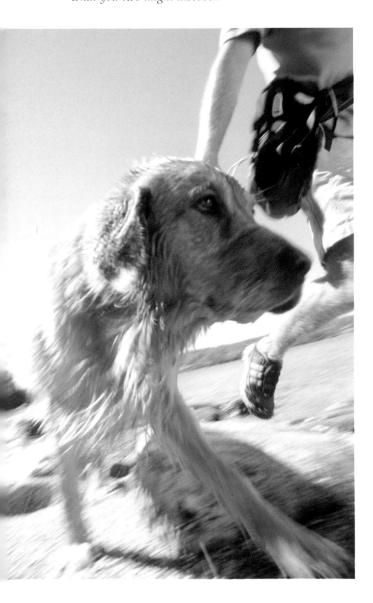

greater freedom of travel. With infants, a front-facing carrier is best. Once a baby can lift his or her head, you can use the backcarrier. Just make sure that it fits properly and that you tighten the shoulder straps.

### Walking with a dog

Your four-legged companion can either be the highlight or the bane of your walking program. A well-trained dog is a joy to walk with. He will heel on the leash, and with the leash handle looped loosely around your wrist, you should be able to swing your arm quite naturally. Your dog offers companionship and added protection, and the enjoyment your pet will get from the additional exercise will be motivation enough for you to walk every day.

If your dog is a "puller," however, your gait will be severely compromised and any hope of maintaining that all-important posture can be forgotten. If this is the case, you might want to walk your dog in open areas where he can safely be let off the leash. This will give you the chance to really "go for it" on your walk.

Make sure, too, that you and your dog are compatible walking companions. If you're very active and regularly walk 5 miles (8 km) five times a week, then a small dog with short legs is going to hold you back; and a large, energetic dog won't be satisfied with a leisurely 20-minute walk around the block.

### Correcting posture problems

Perfect posture relies on symmetry. If there are imbalances in your walk, this can lead to injury. Podiatrists can recommend a technical shoe store where you can get corrective shoes or soles that fit into your existing shoes.

Other posture problems can result if one leg is longer than the other or from a slightly twisted or curved spine, which can cause pain in your hip or knee joints. Look at the hard soles of an old pair of shoes; if the soles are worn more on one side than the other, then you pronate when you walk, meaning your feet turn in or out. If one sole is more worn than the other, this could indicate that your stride is uneven. Again, see a podiatrist for advice.

## How to breathe

Oxygen is the body's most vital need. The human body can survive several days without water and much longer without food, but only a few minutes without oxygen. For many of us, our sedentary lifestyles mean that we take in the minimum amount of oxygen we need for survival and to perform basic activities. Our lungs aren't used to capacity and the muscles involved in their expansion are rarely stretched.

At rest, most sedentary people fill their lungs with about 14 fl oz (400 ml) of air. With exercise, this can increase to 7 pt (4 l) or more—a tenfold increase. If the exercise is regular, the lungs will gradually stretch so that they can take in more air even when at rest. As you become more fit, your body will be able to use oxygen more efficiently.

### Fill your lungs

*As you exert yourself, you'll need to breathe more deeply to give your body the extra oxygen it requires.*

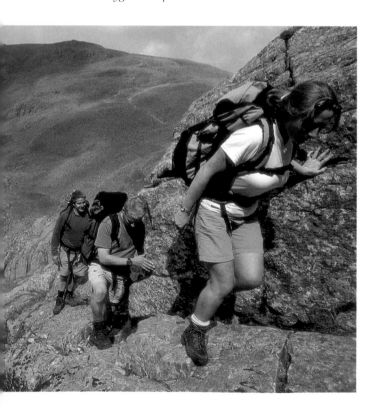

### *The way it works*

The air that we breathe is a mixture of 79 percent nitrogen, around 21 percent oxygen, and 0.03 percent carbon dioxide. As we breathe, the air travels through the mouth, into the throat, down tubes that lead to the lungs called bronchi, and finally into tiny sacs deep in the lungs called alveoli. These alveoli are surrounded by blood vessels, and their thin walls allow the oxygen in the air to diffuse into the blood. Through the bloodstream, the oxygen is delivered to the brain and other organs and to the working muscles. Here the oxygen is used to "burn" fat for fuel. This whole system of supplying energy is known as the aerobic system.

Our bodies have two other energy systems that can supply the working muscles with fuel: the creatine phosphate system and the anaerobic system. In the former, the body uses the high-energy storage molecule creatine in the muscles as a fuel. This molecule can supply the body with a large amount of energy quickly, but only for a short time, like the battery in your car.

The anaerobic system, in which the body uses carbohydrate rather than fat as a fuel source, also provides a quick, short spurt of energy. One of its by-products, however, is lactic acid in the working muscle. An accumulation can lead to cramps. If you do get cramps, this is an indication that you're either not taking in enough oxygen for your body's needs or that your body is unable to supply the muscles with oxygen fast enough. The answer: Slow down and breathe.

### *Breathe deeply*

Walking is an aerobic exercise, and breathing correctly when you walk is all about providing your working muscles with sufficient amounts of oxygen to meet their demands. Many of us do not breathe deeply enough when we exercise. Strolling or walking slowly does not place a great deal of extra demand on the body, but as soon as you start to increase your pace, you'll find that your breathing becomes deeper and heavier. At this point, it's very important to ensure that the maximum amount of oxygen is getting deep into your lungs, because this is where the alveoli are

## BREATHING BETTER

### Belly breathe
*Try to expand your stomach when you breathe in, so you're breathing from your belly. This will maximize the amount of air flowing into your lungs.*

### Count it out
*If you count as you breathe, this will help you find a comfortable rhythm. Try counting 1, 2, 3, 4 on the in breath, and 1, 2, 3 on the out breath.*

### Breathe in step
*Coordinate each breath with your steps. At a fast pace, try one breath in and out for each step.*

### Chant a mantra
*If you're trying to shed weight, chant a mantra such as "I can lose it. Yes, I can!" with your in and out breaths to establish your rhythm and remind you of why you've taken up walking.*

located. If you're breathing too fast or too shallow, then you may be filling the throat and bronchi with air, but not the vital air sacs.

Many people, when told to inhale as much as possible, suck in the stomach and expand the chest. However, it's actually better to "belly breathe," by expanding the stomach as your lungs fill with air. Try it both ways and you'll see the difference.

Many books recommend that you breathe in through your nose and out through the mouth. Taking in air through your nose means it's moistened, warmed and "filtered" by the hairs in your nostrils, all of which make it easier to breathe. Some athletes use a sticky strip across the nose to spread their nostrils and draw more air into their lungs. Short of swallowing the occasional fly, however, there's nothing wrong with breathing through your mouth. Your aim is to maximize oxygen intake in the way that comes naturally, remembering to belly breathe when possible.

### Your natural rhythm
With gentler types of walking, you may not even be aware of how quickly you're breathing. It's often only as you start to really exert yourself that you employ a particular rhythm. To ensure that you are taking in enough air, you can consciously adopt a rhythm by

counting or breathing with your steps. Make sure, however, you do not get out of breath, as the chances are you'll no longer be working aerobically.

As well as helping you get sufficient oxygen, concentrating on the rhythm of your breaths is a way of fixing and calming your mind and can be very therapeutic. Awareness of your breathing is a major feature of many meditation techniques (see page 58).

### Preventing side stitches
Breathing rhythmically also can help relieve these sharp pains just beneath the rib cage, caused by a muscle cramp in the diaphragm. When we breathe in, the diaphragm is pressed down and when we exhale, it moves up. If you've eaten just before walking or you're pushing yourself too hard, this puts extra pressure on the diaphragm and a side stitch may result. Breathing controls the movement of your diaphragm, so changing its pattern can bring relief. Try the following:
- **Breathe deeply** This will stretch the diaphragm.
- **Exhale strongly** Try this when the foot on the opposite side to the stitch hits the floor.
- **Hold your breath** Take a quick breath and hold it for a couple of seconds to force the diaphragm down. Exhale through pursed lips to restrict outward airflow.

## How fast should you walk?

The speed of your walk can play a big part in determining the efficiency of your walking program. If you're trying to improve your fitness, your aim will be to gradually increase your speed as you walk. It's one of the ways that you can push your body a little farther each time and improve your fitness.

What speed should be your goal? This will vary greatly from individual to individual. After you have perfected your technique, the important thing is to start at a pace that is suited to your current level of fitness. The "average" walking speed has been defined as 4 mph on a route of 1 mile (6.5 km/h on a route of 1.6 km). This works out to 1 mile (1.6 km) every 15 minutes. However, most people would find it hard to maintain this pace for a longer distance or on uneven terrain. If 1 mph (1.6 km/h) is all you can manage, that's where you should start. The key is to walk fast without overexertion.

### Stride length and frequency

When walking, the length of your stride should feel natural and not a strain in any way. You should be able to adopt the correct walking posture without undue effort. Some people may feel that their speed is limited by their physical makeup. This is true to a certain extent. Your walking speed is a result of two things: your stride length and frequency.

Your stride length is the more difficult factor to change. It's largely determined by the length of your legs, the flexibility of your hamstring muscles at the backs of your thighs, the amount of rotation around your hip joints, and the flexibility of the tendons and muscles around your hips. Some of these factors you can't change, and attempts to increase your stride length beyond your body's natural range of movement would probably lead to an unnatural, bouncing walk, which would place a significant amount of stress and strain on your joints.

If your short stride lengths are the result of tight hamstring muscles, you can bring improvements by increasing flexibility. Your hamstrings may be tight because you are unused to exercise or simply because you are getting older—tight hamstrings are responsible for the shuffling walk of older people. The more you walk and stretch your muscles, the more flexible you will become and the easier walking will be. Alternatively, your shorter stride lengths could be a result of being overweight. But, again, this can be improved as you walk more and lose weight.

---

**STRIDE LENGTH | explained**

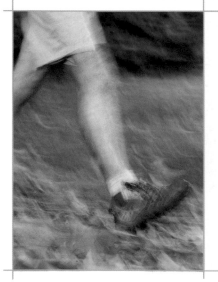

In any group of people walking together, it's not long before you hear the complaint: "I'll never catch up with him. Just look at the length of his legs!" If you find yourself thinking this, then try to remember your basic physics lessons. Think of the leg as a pendulum and remember that the shorter the pendulum, the faster it swings. Therefore, someone with shorter legs can actually walk faster than someone with long legs. If you look at the physique of many racewalkers, they are not unusually tall. If taller people really did have an advantage, you can bet that racewalkers would be built more like basketball players. Good technique will help you increase your stride lengths, as will strong leg muscles. Walking will naturally increase the strength of your legs, and you can try supplementing your walking with resistance exercises in the gym.

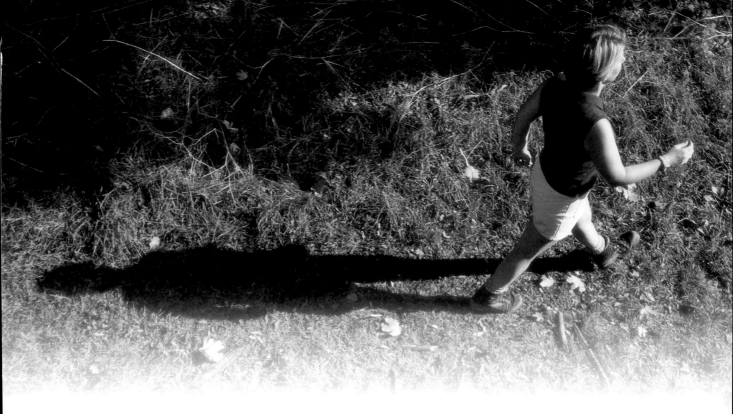

Your stride frequency also can easily be altered. With regular walking, not only will your leg muscles become stronger, but they also can contract at a faster rate. Even if you have short legs, with enough practice you can achieve good walking speeds by increasing your stride frequency.

**A natural stride**
*Keep every part of your body relaxed, focus straight ahead and breathe in rhythm with your stride.*

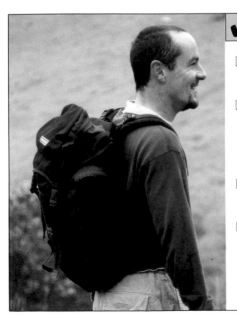

## ✓ ARE YOU READY TO WALK?

❑ **Speed** Start at a pace that's natural for you, and increase the speed gradually so that you are slightly out of breath.

❑ **Stride** Always maintain a comfortable length and frequency. As your hamstrings lengthen, your joints will become more flexible, as your weight begins to fall, you can increase your stride length and therefore your speed.

❑ **Breathing** Breathe from your belly, inhaling through your nose and exhaling through your mouth.

❑ **Posture** Make sure you're walking with correct posture throughout your body. A backpack should sit high on your back, with the straps tightened to keep it level and prevent jostling.

# WARM UP AND COOL DOWN

*No matter the stage you start your walking, warming up
and cooling down are habits you should acquire early.
As you increase the pace and intensity of your walks,
stretching will become even more important.*

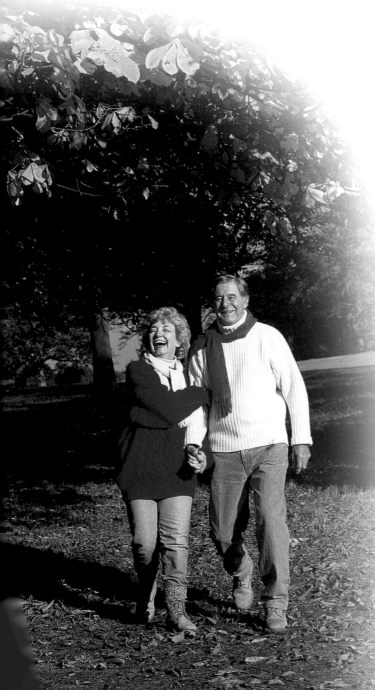

Unless you're about to embark on or have just finished some very vigorous uphill walking or a racewalk, the warm-up and cool-down stages of your walk need not be complicated or take very long. These stages, however, play a vital role in your walking program, helping your body cope with the demands of exercise, preventing strains and injuries, and improving your flexibility.

## Why warm up?

Have you ever driven your car without oil or tried starting it in third gear? If you have, then you're familiar with the awful grinding or the awful bucking that goes with it. The body is not so different. Before you do any exercise, your joints need lubricating with their own internal oil, called synovial fluid, and the body needs to be taken gently "through the gears" so that it can perform comfortably and efficiently.

The warm-up means exactly what it says: raising the body's temperature in preparation for exercise. As the body gets warmer, hormones that dilate the blood vessels are released, enabling more blood to be transported to the working muscles and away from the internal organs. The same hormones act on your heart's natural pacemaker to increase the frequency

### Warm for your warm-up
*Keep your muscles warm when you're
preparing for your walk; particularly
your extremities, which are vulnerable
to cold. Wear layers that can be
removed as body temperature rises.*

> *"An early-morning walk is a*
> *blessing for the whole day."*

### HENRY DAVID THOREAU

and force of its beat, again so more oxygen-rich blood is delivered to the muscles.

With the rise in body temperature, the synovial fluid between the joints becomes less sticky, allowing parts in the joints to glide more easily against each other. This means you're less likely to injure yourself. The colder the weather, the longer this process takes. The increased body temperature also makes the muscles and tendons more elastic (see box, below).

It can be tempting to think of a warm-up as "wasting time" before your workout, particularly if you're busy. Why not just get on with the walk, when you'll be working you body hardest? But skimping on the warm-up is never a good idea. You risk injury and you won't get the most out of your walk.

*Walkers' tips*

## WARMING UP

### Don't push it
*You should feel comfortable and relaxed. Use easy movements and don't rush. This is not the time to be working up a sweat.*

### Prepare mentally
*Use your warm-up as an opportunity to think about what you want to achieve from your walk and your day in general.*

### Focus on your body
*Think about the changes that are occurring internally as you warm up. Feel your heart rate increasing, your joints loosening up and your breathing becoming deeper.*

### Keep covered
*You should be warm during your warm-up, so wear several layers of clothing if you need to. You can always remove these layers later on.*

## MUSCLE FIBERS | explained

Consider a stick of chewing gum. Before you've put it in your mouth, it's stiff, and can easily be ripped in half. Now imagine the same piece of gum once you've been chewing it for several minutes and it has warmed up in your mouth: It's stretchy and pliable, and you can pull it to long lengths before it breaks. Your muscle fiber is very similar to the gum. If you try to exercise while it's cold or before you've warmed up, it may be stiff and prone to damage. Warm the muscles up, and you'll find they can be stretched much farther. This is particularly important on cold days, when the outside temperature makes your muscle fiber less stretchy than normal. Keep extra layers of clothing on until you feel physically warm and your heart is beating faster, delivering warm blood to the working muscle.

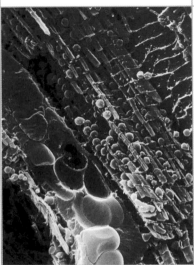

### How to warm up

There are two elements that you should include in every warm-up: mobilization exercises, which loosen up the joints, and gentle activity. The optional part of the warm-up is stretching, which should never be confused with or replace the warm-up.

You can start with the mobilization exercises before you leave the house, or perform them as you walk along (see below). Gentle activity simply means starting off your walk at a slower pace than you'll be walking for the main section of your walk so that you can take your body gradually "up through the gears," lessening the risk of injury. If you do have a tendency to "go for it" as soon as you start off, try to resist this temptation. A more gentle initial pace will increase your body temperature slowly, and give your muscles and tendons time to adapt to the demands being made on them. The warm-up phase of your walk should take about 5 minutes if you're fit or 10 to 15 minutes if you haven't exercised for a while.

## Loosening up

*The mobilization exercises loosen up the muscles you're about to use. You can do them before you set out, or do the upper-body exercises as you walk along and stop briefly to loosen your legs and feet. Then you're ready to continue with the gentle exercise phase.*

Start at the top. Breathe out and consider your facial expression. Are you frowning? Are your teeth clenched? Relax and prepare to enjoy your walk.

**a** Lift your shoulders toward your ears, and then lower.

**b** Bend the head to one side, letting your ear drop gently toward your shoulder. Hold for 5 to 10 seconds, then drop the head toward the other shoulder. Next, look down and drop your chin to your chest. Avoid moving the head backward or rolling it around; this compresses the vertebrae in your neck. Lift your shoulders again, then circle them a few times.

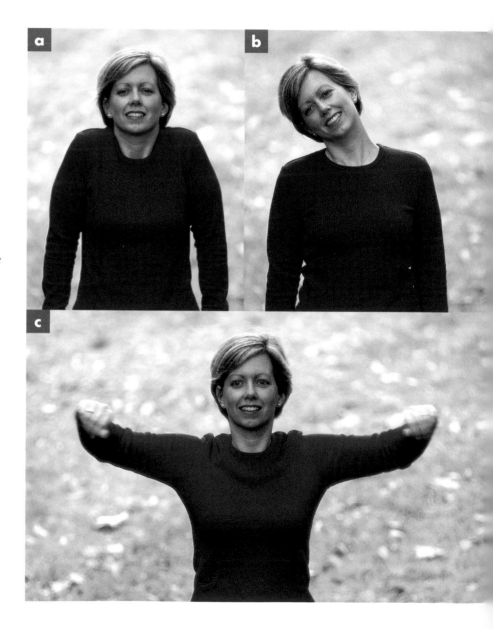

## To stretch or not to stretch?

Although an essential part of any cool-down routine (see page 38), there's some controversy about whether stretches should be included in the warm-up. Recent studies have suggested that stretching before exercise may not bring any more benefit than mobilization exercises and gentle activity. Other experts maintain that preexercise stretches are a desirable part of your warm-up, because they help to prevent injury, and improve flexibility and motion around a joint.

The answer is to do what you feel is right for you, as long as you bear in mind the following two points: Never stretch a cold muscle and always make sure that you're performing the stretches correctly. If you do decide to include stretches in your warm-up, use the techniques shown on pages 40 and 41. Hold each for at least 10 seconds and, if you're short of time, focus on the leg stretches.

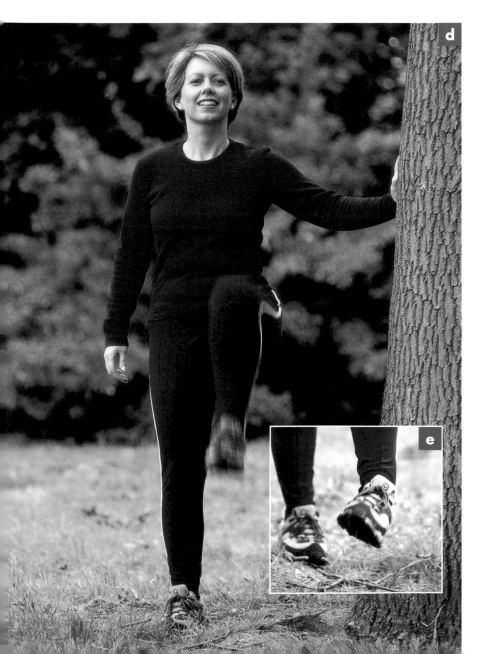

**c** Circle the arms, keeping them slightly bent. Make progressively larger and larger circles, but always controlled—don't fling the arms. If you feel self-conscious, you may be more comfortable doing these indoors. As you circle, practice your "belly breathing" (see page 31), inhaling as you raise your arms and exhaling as you lower them. Make sure you breathe deeply, expanding your belly as you inhale and sucking it in gently as you exhale.

**d** Lean against a wall or tree for support and lift one knee as high as you can, then the other. Lift the first knee again. Point and flex the foot a few times.

**e** Circle the foot at the ankle. Repeat with the other foot.

## The purpose of the cool-down

As you exercise, your heart rate increases and your heart beats more forcefully. When you're ready to stop, it's necessary to give your body time to return to normal. The cool-down is an essential part of any physical activity program. It involves gradually reducing the heart rate and breathing, and stretching the muscles to maintain or develop flexibility. During your cool-down, your blood is routed away from your working muscles and back to your internal organs. Your blood temperature will drop and your breathing will slow. The more fit you become, the more quickly your body will return to its normal state.

As the blood is pumped around your body, it's assisted by a milking-like action in the muscles. The gastrocnemius—the largest calf muscle—is particularly important in this respect—so much so that it's called the "second heart." Each time these muscles contract as you walk, they help move the blood up your legs. If you suddenly stop walking and the muscles stop their action, the blood tends to pool in the lower legs,

resulting in an inadequate supply of blood to the brain. It's not uncommon for people to feel faint or even pass out if they suddenly stop exercising. If you need to stop when you're out walking, make sure you keep your feet moving by marching in place or even just lifting your heels off the ground.

### How to cool down

There are two elements in every cool-down: reduced-intensity activity and stretches. Just like starting your walk with gentle activity, reducing the intensity at the end simply involves walking slower than normal for 5 to 10 minutes. Use this period to reflect on your walk, what you've achieved, and what you'd like to do next time. Once you've stopped, you can begin your stretching routine, as outlined on the following pages.

### Why stretch?

Most experts agree that being physically fit is about more than just reducing your risk of heart attack. You may end up at the age of 80 with the heart of a

## FLEXIBILITY *for health*

▶ If you regularly stretch the muscles that attach to the pelvis—the hamstrings, hip flexors and quadriceps—you'll reduce the stress placed on the lower back.

▶ Stretching exercises that emphasize flexibility have been shown to increase ankle, knee joint, and lower-back flexibility in older adults.

▶ A safe stretch is one that is gentle. If a stretch hurts, stop doing it.

▶ Muscles that are warm from jogging, cycling, or other aerobic exercise can stretch farther and more safely.

▶ Stretching increases the supply of blood and nutrients to your joints, so reducing your risk of joint degeneration.

▶ By realigning soft tissue structure, stretching helps you achieve good posture and balance.

*"After a day's walk, everything has twice its usual value."*

GEORGE MACAULEY TREVELYAN

*English historian*

50-year-old by doing lots of aerobic activities, but if you're not strong or flexible, your quality of life may be severely compromised. Studies have shown that the strength of your grip—an indicator of general muscle strength—is a very strong predictor of independence in older age. Walking will help maximize your muscle strength—for upper-body exercises, see page 181. But flexibility also plays a crucial part in determining your ability to stay active and independent.

Much of your flexibility is genetically determined; the way your skeleton is constructed and the positioning and range of movement of your joints also have an influence. Also, the older you get and the less you use your muscles and tendons, the more they tighten. Tightened muscles and tendons lead to poor posture—for example, tight chest and shoulder muscles lead to rounded shoulders (see also page 32).

The good news is that problems such as soreness and muscle pulls or strains appear to be lower in people who maintain good flexibility.

## Safe stretching

Following all the safety guidelines outlined on the following pages, stretching is safe and beneficial for most people. It can be particularly helpful for those who suffer from back or neck pain, as it relieves tension and improves posture. If you do suffer from pain in these areas, you should, however, consult a doctor before taking up any new form of exercise. He or she will be able to advise on stretching techniques specifically suited to your condition.

Stretching is also beneficial for those recovering from injury. This is because muscle damage causes fibrous scar tissue to form in the muscle. This hard tissue does not stretch very easily, and so can lessen the flexibility in the muscle, increasing the risk of future injury. Once the muscle has started to heal, stretching can help loosen it up again. A qualified fitness instructor or physiotherapist will be able to advise on the best stretching techniques for you.

*Walkers' tips*

## EFFECTIVE STRETCHING

**Stretch regularly**
*Use stretches as part of every cool-down, and pause to stretch during your walk if you feel any tension or muscle soreness.*

**Consider the whole body**
*Mix upper-body stretches with calf, hamstring, quad and shin stretches.*

**Know your level**
*Leave more time for stretching if you are new to regular exercise.*

**Concentrate**
*Ignore the looks of passers-by as you do your stretches. Focus on your technique.*

**Stay in a natural range**
*Avoid stretching your joints in a direction in which they would not normally move.*

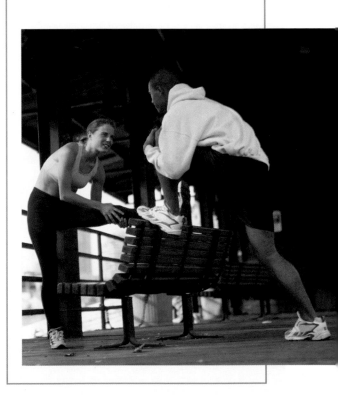

## Flexibility stretches

The following stretches focus on the major muscles you use while walking, and will help to improve your flexibility and stride length. None require workout machines or special gear, so they can be done outside. These stretches are an optional part of your warm-up routine, but should be included in every cool-down (see page 38). Hold each stretch 10 to 30 seconds, then release gently. Never bounce a stretch; it can lead to injury.

## The calves

*When walking, more than three-quarters of your forward propulsion comes from your calf muscles* (gastrocnemii), *so it's especially important to stretch them after walking.*

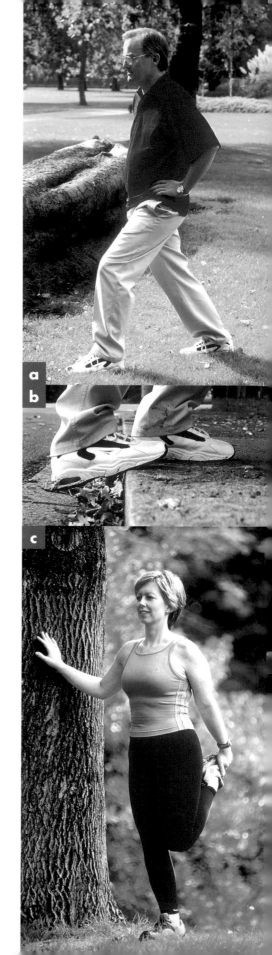

Stand with your legs hip-width apart and take one step back.
**a** Bend at the knee with the other leg but not past your ankle. Keep your back leg straight and your heel pushed down. Check that your toes are pointing forward, not out to the side. You should feel the stretch along the calf of this back leg. Hold, then repeat this stretch on the other leg.

**b** *Alternatively:* A more intense stretch can be achieved by using a step or the street curb. Stand on the top edge of the curb with your back to the street. Step back and rest the ball of your foot on the step or curb, hanging your heel off the edge. Push down into the heel to stretch your calf. Lean the body slightly forward for balance. Hold, then repeat on the other leg.

## The fronts of the thighs

*If your legs are aching after a walk, it's often around the fronts of your thighs* (quadriceps). *A good stretch of your quadriceps as you're cooling down can prevent stiffness.*

**c** Place your right hand on a fence, tree or wall for support. Bend your left knee and grasp the foot behind you with your left hand. Slowly and gently bend your leg up behind you as far as is comfortable. Keep your supporting leg slightly bent so that your knee

is not locked in the straight position. As you hold the stretch you'll feel the tension in the front of your thigh. Make sure that you keep both knees close to each other and push your hips forward. Hold, then release slowly. Repeat with the right leg.

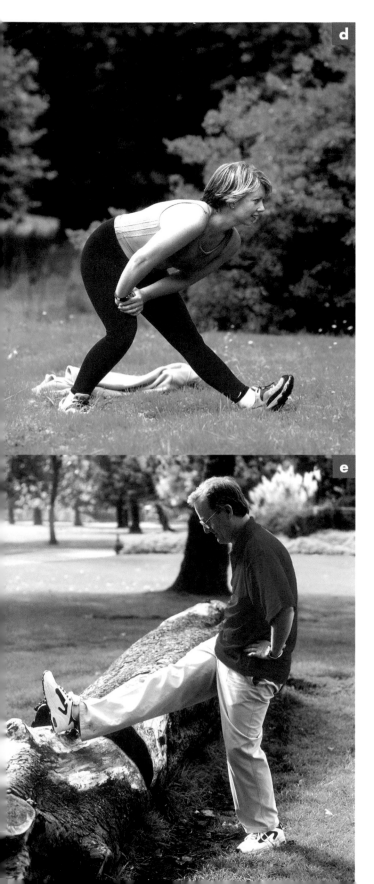

### SAFETY FIRST

If you're unsure whether you're performing the stretches correctly, it's probably better not to do them at all. If you have poor balance or coordination, you may put yourself at risk of falling or straining a muscle or joint. The risk of injury from a poorly performed stretch far outweighs the risk of injury from not stretching. If you get a chance, seek advice from a professional fitness instructor and ask him or her to observe your stretching technique and correct you if necessary.

## The backs of the thighs

*Your hamstrings play a big part in determining your stride length and your posture (see page 32), so make sure that you stretch them sufficiently after every walk.*

**d** Take one step forward about 2 ft (60 cm) with your left leg. Place that heel on the ground, with your toes pointing upward. Bend your right knee and rest your hands on your thigh. Now lean over your straight left leg. Stick your butt out and keep your back flat and your head looking forward. You should feel the stretch in the left leg from your butt through to the back of your knee. Hold, then repeat on the right leg.

**e** *Alternatively:* Use a log, park bench, or another prop to elevate the straight leg. Perform the stretch as above, and bring the upper body forward to achieve a more intense stretch. Hold, then repeat the stretch on the other leg.

## The shins

*The muscles at the fronts of the shins (tibialis anterior) are used a great deal in walking but are often neglected during stretching. This can lead to strains or other injuries, such as shinsplints (see pages 55 and 113).*

**a** Cross one leg over the other, with the toe of the top foot resting on the ground. Gently bend the supporting leg so that it pushes against the calf of the top leg. You should feel a stretch in the shin of the top leg. Hold, then repeat with the other leg. If you find it difficult to balance while performing this stretch, lean on a tree or fence for support.

## Upper body, arms and shoulders

*This stretch is good if you've been increasing the intensity of your walk by pumping your arms, have included upper-body strength exercises, or are feeling tense from carrying a day pack.*

**b** Stand with your legs hip-width apart and the knees slightly bent. Reach above the head with both arms and grasp the hands together. Turn the palms skyward and push up without locking the elbows. Imagine that your belly button is attached to the lower part of your spine, and pull in your stomach, without arching the back. Hold, then release.

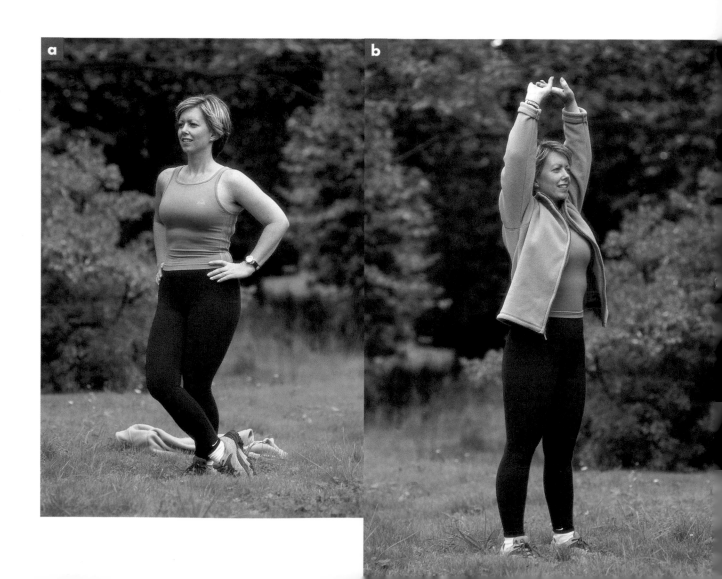

## The chest

*Another stretch that works your upper body, this targets the muscles that power your arm swing.*

**c** Hold your hands together behind your back, with the elbows slightly bent. Slowly raise the arms as far as is comfortable, without leaning forward or arching your lower back. You should feel a stretch across the front of your chest. Hold, then release.

**d** *Alternatively:* If your chest and shoulders are not very flexible, and you can't grasp your hands at the back, simply stretch your arms behind you with the palms facing. Hold a few seconds, then repeat.

### ✓ SAFE TO STRETCH?

❑ **Check your technique** Are you performing the stretches correctly? If you're unsure don't stretch.

❑ **Know your limits** Stretch the muscle as far as you can without causing pain. If it hurts, stop.

❑ **Don't bounce** Move into each stretch gradually and hold steady for 10 to 30 seconds.

❑ **Stretch when warm** Perform 5 to 10 minutes of gentle exercise to warm up before you stretch.

❑ **Balance your stretches** If you do an exercise on one leg, make sure you do it on the other.

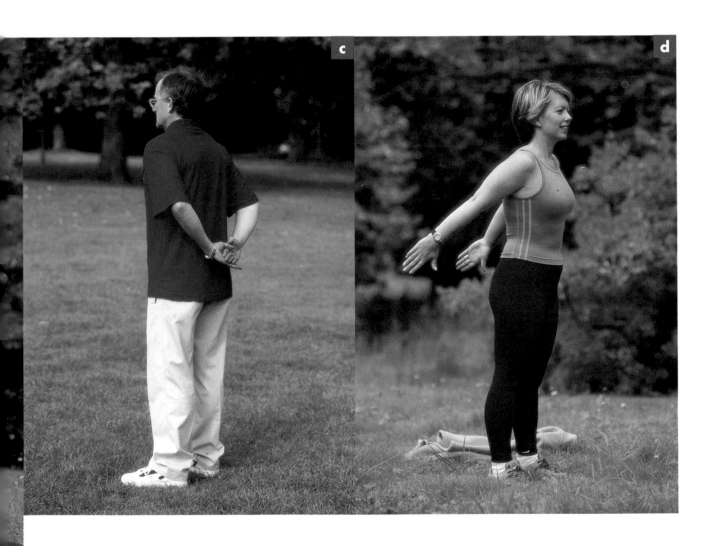

# WORKING **HARDER**

*A major principle of any exercise program is the concept of "overload." This means pushing your body just that little bit farther each time you exercise in order to improve your performance.*

Overload is all about making your heart beat that little bit faster or stronger, or making increased demands on your muscles by asking them to contract more forcefully or more rapidly. Weight lifters progressively add more weight to improve their strength and increase the size of their muscles. The same principle applies to everyone who exercises, whatever the type of exercise he or she is doing. If you increase the demands you make on your body you'll be rewarded with stronger muscles. Don't forget that the heart is a muscle, too, and it will respond to overload in the same way as the other muscles in your body.

If you stick to your walking plan, it will start to bring results: Your breathing will become less labored; you'll find that you have more of a spring in your step and you'll be less tired at the end of your walk. At this stage, you're ready to kick things up a notch and introduce overload into your program. There are three ways of doing this. You can increase the duration, frequency or intensity of your walks. These factors can be used individually or combined, depending on what you want from your walk. Intensity can be achieved in many ways, such as walking faster, adding resistance, using your arms more and tackling hills.

*Walkers' tips*

### LIFESTYLE WALKING

**Use the stairs**
*If you live in an apartment or work in a office building, forget the elevator and take the stairs instead. If you have a sedentary job, go find the colleague when you need to discuss something rather than call on the phone.*

**Go on foot**
*If you would normally drive to see a friend or neighbor, walk instead.*

**Take the long way**
*If your local store is close by, extend the route to give yourself some extra walking time.*

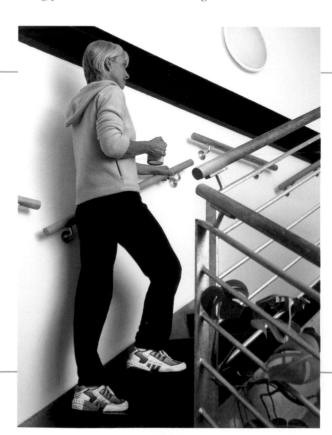

## Walk for longer

"Lack of time" is the most common reason cited for not exercising. If time is the main barrier that prevents you from walking, then increasing the duration of your walks may sound difficult. But is this a real or perceived barrier? Many people find that as they progress through their walking programs, time becomes less of an issue. As they start to enjoy walking more, they make the time in their day for it.

But if you're new to walking, don't worry if you really can't take additional time out of your schedule. As you become more fit, you'll complete the same walk in less time. If you can still devote the same amount of time to your walk, then try walking a little farther. Leave out a shortcut, or double back on a section of the walk. Also try increasing the intensity of your walk. You can also increase the total length of time you spend walking by including several short walks in your day. Two or three 10-minute exercise sessions add to your overall time spent walking and are easy to build

into your daily routine: Take a walk at lunchtime; use the stairs instead of the elevator; deliver a message personally; or get off the bus a stop early and walk the rest of the way. This will all combine to help you to achieve your goals.

## Walk more often

Increasing the frequency of your walks can go hand-in-hand with increasing their length. By adding short walks to your day, you will, of course, be walking more often. More frequent walking may be the solution if you can't find large chunks of time on a regular basis. Exercise must be regular to get the best results, and three half-hour walks in one week should bring you more benefit than one three-hour walk a week.

## Step up the pace

The intensity of your walks is determined by how much energy you expend with each step. The easiest way to increase intensity is to walk faster. If you want to step it up a little, consider varying the conditions of your walk (see page 46), using your arms and/or poles (see page 50), or stepping up the pace to a walk-run technique (see page 52).

Increased pace should be your aim for every walk and one of the major variables in your walking program. Time your usual walk, and then resolve to do it a few minutes faster. Or let another walker set the pace; if you see someone in the distance, try to pass him or her. Alternatively, start to walk with someone who you think is a little more fit than you. You'll have a companion and will encourage each other.

Increase your pace only after you've mastered a near-perfect walking technique and can maintain good posture. Speeding up with poor technique can lead to injury. As you walk faster, you'll need to lean forward slightly to keep your balance. Focus on contracting muscles; it will feel like your legs are stiffening, but it will shorten your stride and make your legs move faster. Allow this to happen, but make sure you're walking comfortably and not bouncing.

### Stop early
*Get off the bus or subway one or two stops before your final destination and walk the rest of the way.*

### Walk to school
*Accompany your kids in the morning. This will give you a boost of energy at the start of your day. Walk at a fairly fast pace once you're on your own.*

### Create a good habit
*Walk at the same time each day so that it becomes a part of your regular routine. Good habits can be just as hard to break as bad ones.*

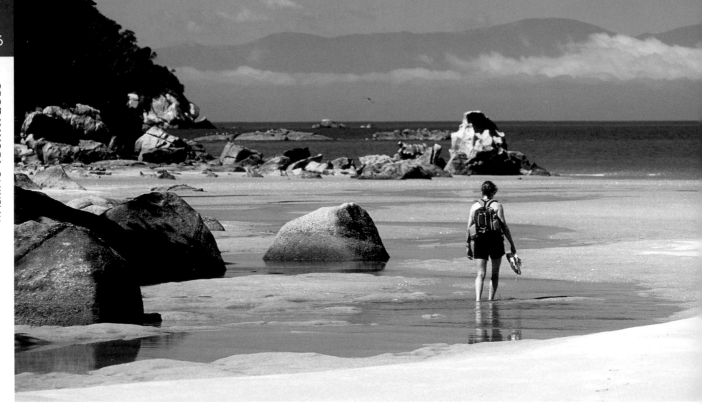

## Adding resistance

If you want to increase the intensity of your walks as well as add a bit of variety, start investigating other routes. Walking in conditions different from the usual will challenge your body in new ways, particularly if you plan a route that covers challenging terrain. Increase intensity in natural ways by walking on sand, snow, and against the wind. Artificial means include apparatus such as treadmills and stair-climbers.

### Footprints in the sand

Walking on either a level paved surface or a grass track requires similar energy. Walking on sand, however, will make you work much harder. Because the sand absorbs the downward motion you generate with each step, you need more energy to lift your foot again. Walking on soft snow is three times more demanding than walking on pavement. Make sure you are prepared when investigating new areas (see pages 68 to 81).

### A walk in the wind

We've all walked in conditions when every step seems to be a battle with Mother Nature. This is often the case with wind. Walking against a head wind is harder than walking in calm conditions. Your body catches the wind and is forced in the other direction. Studies of runners have shown that energy expenditure against a 10 mph (16 km/h) head wind increased by 5 percent compared with a windless day. If you're timing your walk, allow for wind resistance so that you don't become discouraged if you haven't improved. The good news is that you'll benefit more from these windy walks, because your muscles work harder to push your body against the force of the wind, and it can be incredibly invigorating.

### Trying out treadmills

Though you may prefer to walk outside, there are times when the weather, location or personal-safety issues can detract from your enjoyment. Such a time would be a good opportunity to try out a treadmill at your local gym or fitness center. Treadmill walking is a good supplement to your outdoor program, because it allows you to closely monitor and vary your speed, distance and time. If you note and increase these factors over several weeks, you can easily build up the intensity of your walking. Some treadmills allow you to increase your intensity with an uphill option (see page 48), and

### Against the grain

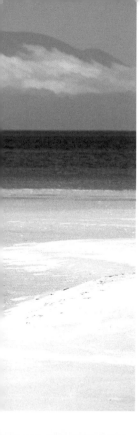

*Beach walking leads to great energy expenditure. Walking on sand takes almost twice the energy as walking on a hard surface or on grass.*

### Blown backward

*Against a strong wind, the energy required to maintain your normal pace increases by around 40 percent.*

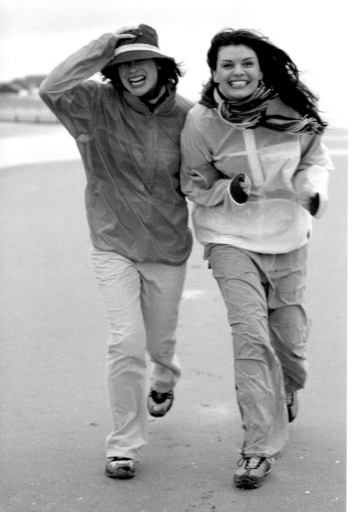

they may also have preset programs, such as "cardiovascular" or "fat-burning" sessions, which automatically change speed and gradient at various intervals as you walk. Some advanced treadmills allow you to monitor your heart rate as you exercise and show you how many calories you're burning. They may also have features such as a springy belt, which provides shock-absorption and helps reduce the pressure on your joints.

Treadmills have many other advantages. Machines are often positioned in front of full-length mirrors, providing a great opportunity for checking your posture. Also, the level walking surface means that you're more likely to put an even amount of weight on each leg, and are less likely to trip or fall.

If you're considering buying a treadmill, look for one with a motor-driven conveyor belt that has speed control, an incline option and good arm rails for safety. Seek professional advice, because good treadmills are costly. You want to be sure you choose the one best for you. The first time you get on a treadmill, you'll need an instructor to show you how to operate the machine and to see that you're walking with the correct posture. Here are some points to bear in mind:

- **Starting off** Stand with your feet straddling the treadmill and set a slow speed of around 2 mph (3.2 km/h). Using the handrails for support, step onto the track and start with a gentle stroll.
- **Increasing the speed** Once you're happy with your start-up pace, begin to increase the speed. When you feel confident, let go of the handrails. Holding on prevents you from pumping your arms, so you're not working as hard as you could be. It may also hamper your walking technique.
- **Check your posture** Walking in place is a great opportunity to think about posture. Working from the feet upward, check that your posture reflects your everyday walking technique (see page 26).
- **Push yourself** If you're not following a preset program, use the manual setting to work at a pace that's fast, but without overexerting. If you find yourself drifting toward the back of the moving track, you may have it set too fast.

### *Walking uphill*

One sure way to increase the intensity of your walk and introduce "overload" is to include an incline or hill. If you're wearing a heart-rate monitor (see page 133), you'll be amazed at just how quickly your heart rate increases as you walk uphill. Moving your own body weight vertically rather than horizontally dramatically increases the load on your muscles and your overall effort level, including how hard your heart is working. The heavier you are, the greater the demands. On steep inclines, it's not unusual for even a fit person's heart rate to increase by about 20 percent.

The average energy expenditure for a person weighing 150 lbs (68.5 kg), walking at 3.5 mph (5.5 km/h) on flat ground is 350 calories per hour. At the same speed on a 4 percent incline, energy expenditure for the same person will be 400 calories per hour, and on a 10 percent incline 500 calories per hour. A 4 percent incline is equivalent to a moderately steep hill, a 10 percent incline a steep hill and a 15 percent incline an extremely steep hill. If you can resist the urge to slow down too much when you hit a gentle hill, you'll be greatly increasing the benefits you get from your walk.

### *Walking down again*

It was long thought that walking downhill expended much less energy than walking on the flat. If this were true, it would mean that adding inclines to your walk would be "negative" work, with the downhill section of the walk simply canceling out the work you had done on the uphill section. We know now, however, that this is not the case. As you walk downhill, your muscles have to work against gravity, contracting to slow down your descent.

On very steep slopes this can be harder work than walking on the flat. But, on the whole, walking downhill expends about the same amount of energy as walking on the flat. This means that the total energy expended on a hilly walk, from both the up and down sections, will usually exceed the amount exerted on the same distance on the flat, so don't be afraid to introduce hills to your walk.

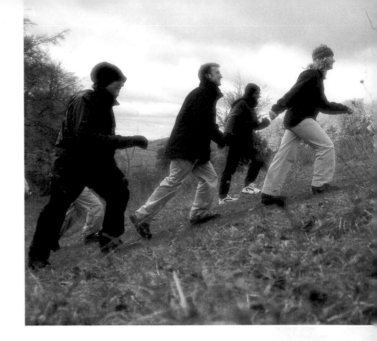

## Tackling hills

Walking up and down hills requires slightly different techniques from those you use for walking on the flat.

**a** When going uphill, it's best to shorten your stride length. **b** Think of the incline as a staircase with risers about 8 in. (20 cm) high. Climbing stairs forces you into a short stride length and makes the quadriceps, the large muscles of your thighs, do most of the hard work. Lean forward slightly to help you to keep your balance. The rule of walking at a pace at which you're not overexerting applies to hills as well as to the flat.

Going down steep slopes can be a strain on fragile knees and hip joints. The added force of gravity can make walking downhill more difficult than uphill walking. **c** Take smaller steps and don't lean backward. Make sure that the knees don't lock by bending them slightly.

**d** If the slope is very steep, take a zigzag course, or switchbacks, in the same way that a mountain road goes side to side, rather than straight down the mountain.

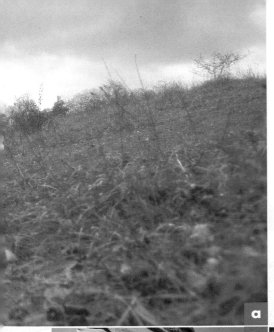

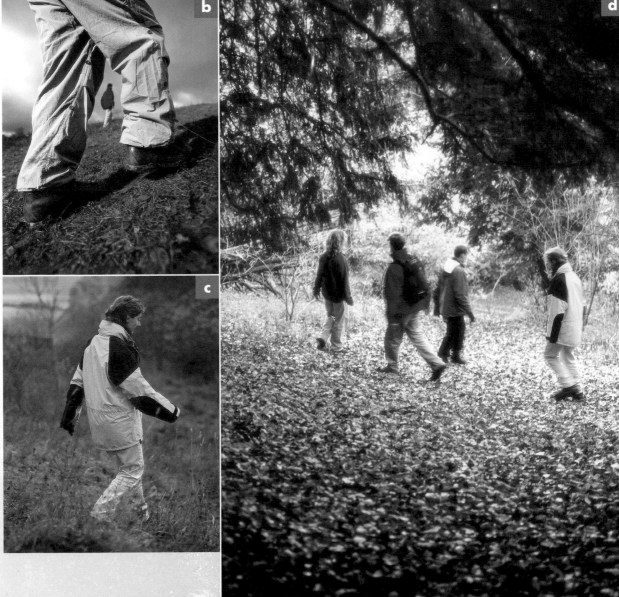

## Using your arms and poles

There's no reason why your walks should work only the muscles in your legs and lower body. If you want to get more benefit from each walk without walking for longer or farther, then concentrate on your arms and the way you use them. Whether you simply swing them with more force and control or you decide to use poles, the work of your arms, shoulders and upper body makes your heart beat faster and your body burn more calories. The extra movement should also improve your strength in these muscles.

Some people believe that adding weights to their ankles or carrying weights will increase the intensity of their walk. While it's true to say that a fit, well-trained walker in laboratory conditions will expend more energy using weights, the real world is somewhat different. Carrying weights affects a walker's natural gait. In addition, weights can cause joint problems in the elbows and shoulders by placing stress at these points as the arms swing. But perhaps the biggest

problem with weights is that they feel unnatural and cumbersome, and they can hamper your enjoyment of walking. One of the delights of walking is the feeling of freedom that comes with it. The idea that you don't need to load yourself down with equipment to take part in the activity is one of walking's greatest appeals. You can increase the intensity of your walk in much safer and more comfortable ways than by carrying weights. Concentrate, instead, on increasing your walking speed or adding intensity with a hill. Or, if you want to use your arms more, focus on your swing or try using poles.

### Strengthen your swing

The simplest way to bring your arms into play is to change the way you move them. Make sure that you've adopted the general arm position described on page 27, with the arms bent at 90 degrees, and move your arms briskly and with controlled, definite movements. This arm action is great if you are trying to increase

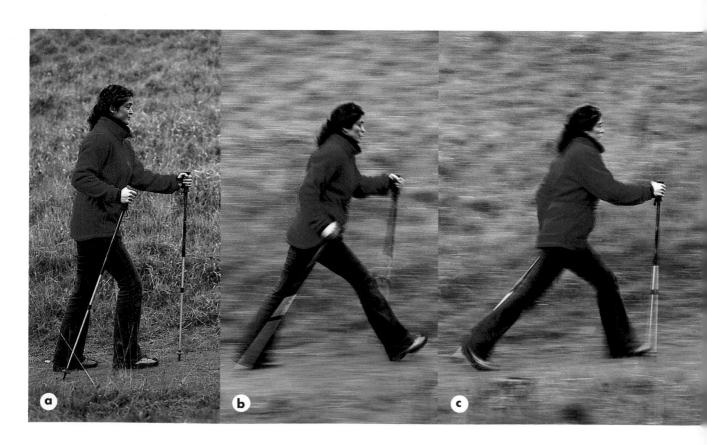

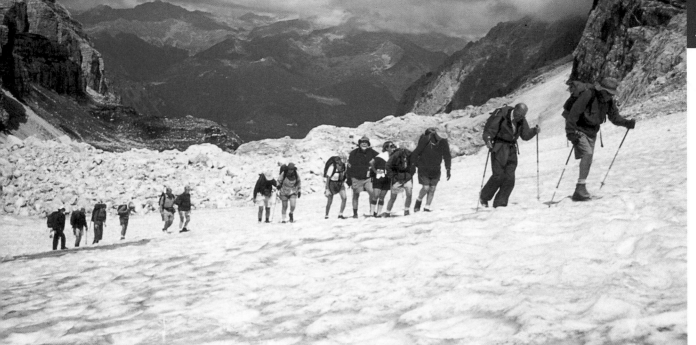

### Double intensity

*As well as increasing energy expenditure, poles are a useful aid to balance on demanding walks.*

## POLE TECHNIQUE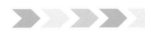

Using trekking poles should enhance, rather than replace, your normal walking technique, so allow the poles to swing in the same relaxed, fluid rhythm your arms would naturally adopt. Hold the poles close to your body, with your hands through the wrist straps, and keep a loose grip on the handles **a.** Strike the ground with your leading foot, then bring the opposite pole forward, planting it in the ground in line with your leading foot **b.** Use this pole to propel yourself forward, allowing it to rest on the wrist straps as it swings forward. Remember to push back on the pole, not down on it, with the tip pointing back. As your trailing foot moves to take the lead, swing the pole forward on the opposite side **c.** Hold your shoulders down and keep them relaxed as you walk, moving the poles with a swing of the upper torso and hips.

your speed, because the more vigorously you pump your arms, the faster your feet will follow. Make sure that your arms are moving back and forth not side to side, and that you bring them only to chest height with each swing.

### Using poles

In recent years, more and more people have started to walk with poles. Unlike weights, poles are lightweight enough not to produce an unnatural arm swing. They can significantly increase the energy you expend on your walk by up to 30 percent. This is because, unlike weights, they are used to propel you forward. As you plant your poles and push against them with each step, you create a resistance against the ground. This recruits much more of the muscle mass of your upper body, including the arms, shoulders and chest, which in turn leads to increased energy expenditure. The proper technique does take some perfecting (see box, left), and most poles come with good instructions and sometimes even a video. Bear in mind that poles are best on natural terrain and trails rather than paved surfaces and hard roads, where the impact of planting the pole may jar your shoulder and elbow joints. For more information on buying poles see page 134.

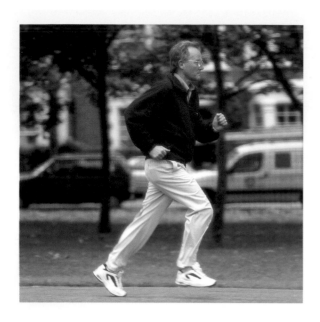

## RUNNING

As with walking, make sure that when you run your posture is good. Think about your posture from the feet upward. Strike the ground with the heel first and follow through to the ball of the foot and the toe. Then push off with the toe. Keep your stomach pulled in, butt tucked under and don't arch your back. Run tall, with a slight lean forward. Bend your arms to a little less than 90° and swing them back and forth straight ahead; avoid crossing them in front of your body. Relax your shoulders and neck. The head should be centered on the shoulders, chin parallel to the ground.

### The walk-run technique

Even when walking is their main activity, some people find that they like to include some running for variety. It's important to stress from the outset that walking is by no means an inferior form of exercise to running. In fact, regular, intense walking can be every bit as demanding as running, though without the risks of injury. That's why more and more top athletes are turning to walking as the best way to keep in shape without the risk of injury. However, as you pick up the pace and start to exceed speeds of 4.5 mph (7 km/h), you may find yourself naturally breaking into a run, and you no longer have one foot touching the ground at all times.

At walking speeds faster than 4.5 mph (7 km/h), running actually becomes more economical. If you do manage to resist the temptation to run at this point, and maintain your walk, you'll be increasing your fitness tremendously. Running seems easier at these speeds because we all have our own natural body "springs" in the arches of the feet. These springs absorb the energy that's pushed into them as the feet hit the ground and then, just like a coiled spring, return that energy to the running legs. As long as your body is up to the extra impact that running places on your ankle,

knee and hip joints, you're at a good level of all-round fitness (see pages 140 to 147), and you've checked out the risks with your doctor if necessary (see page 97), why not incorporate the walk-run technique into your regular program?

If and when your body is ready, let running come naturally. The first urge to start will probably happen on an imperceptibly gentle downhill slope. Running

### TYPICAL TRAINING PROGRAM

| Week | Activity to perform 4 days a week |
|------|-----------------------------------|
| 1 | Run 2 minutes, walk 4 minutes. Repeat 5 times. |
| 2 | Run 4 minutes, walk 2 minutes. Repeat 5 times. |
| 3 | Run 5 minutes, walk 2.5 minutes. Repeat 4 times. |
| 4 | Run 7 minutes, walk 3 minutes. Repeat 3 times. |
| 5 | Run 8 minutes, walk 2 minutes. Repeat 3 times. |

like this can be very exhilarating, and it can ultimately contribute to "overload" (see page 44). Introduce running to your program gradually (see box, below). If your running starts to compromise your walking speed, wait until you're more fit before running again.

When you're planning your walk-run program, you can work out times for each specific section, or base it around specific landmarks on your route. Try the five-week program in the chart, opposite, on Mondays, Wednesdays, Fridays and Saturdays, and taking the other two days off. Each weekly dose gives you a 30-minute total workout per day, and provides a graduated activity by increasing the amount of running time in relation to walking time as the weeks progress.

**SAFETY FIRST**

Don't overdo it, and bear in mind that the walk-run technique is an option. Pushing yourself too hard by trying to run before you're ready may be frustrating and lead to you abandoning your program. Listen to your body and build up gradually, otherwise you may suffer an injury, which could put you months behind in your training program.

## WALK-RUN

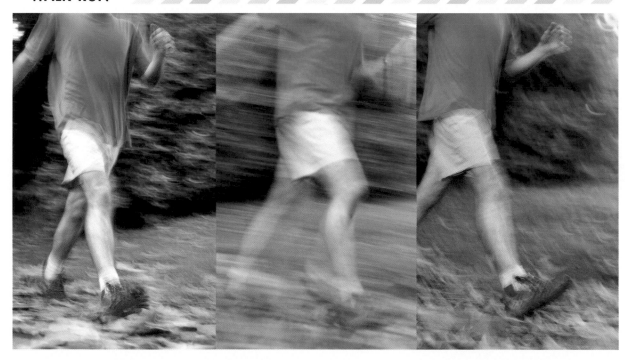

Run for just 1 minute at a time, then walk for a bit, and run again when you feel like it. Try walking between two points, such as streetlights or trees, and then running between the next two, alternating until you've had enough. Make sure that you keep up a good pace, without overdoing it, because this will work your body harder and increase the benefits you get from your exercise. Always include a period of slower exercise toward the end of your walk-run to cool down.

# **TECHNIQUE** TROUBLESHOOTER

*You've started walking, and you're making good progress. However, there are some health concerns that are holding you back. If any of these complaints sound familiar, here are a few solutions.*

**My feet ache after I walk. What could I be doing wrong?**

You must have a good shoe with proper grip and cushioning. When you buy shoes, make sure that you buy them from a reputable store and that they are comfortable. You'll need to change them every 350 miles (560 km), depending on your body weight. See Chapter 5 (pages 124 to 127) for further advice on buying the correct fit.

**I'm worried about getting back pain when I walk. What can I do to avoid it?**

Back pain can be caused by any number of factors, but one of the most common is poor posture. Use the posture guidelines (see page 26) and make sure that you're not hunching your shoulders or arching your back. Get someone to stand in front of you and watch you as you walk, or walk on a treadmill facing the mirror. Tight hamstring muscles can cause lower-back pain, so try to increase your flexibility in these muscles (see page 41). If the pain does not subside after a few days, speak to your doctor.

**I often feel tense and achy in my shoulders and upper back after a walk. Why is this?**

Your upper-body technique may be poor. If your shoulders are hunched and your arms stiff, then you're holding tension and this can lead to muscle soreness. Try to relax, keeping your torso straight but not stiff, and swing your arms naturally. Try not to think of your walk as the next thing that has to be done in your hectic day, but rather as an opportunity to unwind.

**I find it difficult to keep to a regular breathing pattern when walking. What can I do?**

Try to regulate your breathing by counting to 4 as you inhale and to 3 as you exhale, or by coordinating it with your step (see page 31). Remember that you may need to adjust this rhythm if you step up the pace or slow down. Your aim should be to reach a point where you no longer notice your breathing. If you get a stitch, try alternating your breathing pattern (see page 31).

**I'm trying to walk with proper technique but it "feels wrong." What should I change?**

Nothing. If you've been walking incorrectly all your life, then once you adopt good walking technique your body can feel rather different. You're using muscles in a different way and you'll certainly be aware of these changes. The golden rule is that it's only "wrong" if you're in pain. There's no need to change anything unless you feel specific strains that do not go away after a period of rest. If so, check with your doctor.

**I think I have "shinsplints." What are they and how can I avoid them?**

The most common complaint from novice walkers is "shinsplints," an acute pain in the front of the lower leg. During fast walking, the muscles of the shin contract and extend to flex and point the foot. Most people are not accustomed to using these muscles this much and therefore they can become sore and inflamed. If you've spent your life in high heels, then the muscles at the front of the shin have hardly ever had to perform the full range of motion. The pain may subside with rest. If not, see your doctor. Warming up more slowly and making sure you have the right shoes will prevent the condition (see page 113).

**I often get a cramp after a walk. Is there anything I can do to prevent this from happening?**

If you've been for a fairly strenuous walk, it's not uncommon to experience a cramp in your feet, calves or thighs shortly after you finish. This is because of a buildup of lactic acid and other chemicals in the muscles and because of small areas of muscle-fiber damage. Cramps also occur when you sweat excessively, as the loss of sodium from salt disrupts muscle-cell activity. A strenuous walk in hot weather therefore puts you at greatest risk of a cramp. Treat cramps by stretching and massaging the affected muscles (see page 113). Cramps should only last a few minutes. If you experience pain for more than an hour, see your doctor.

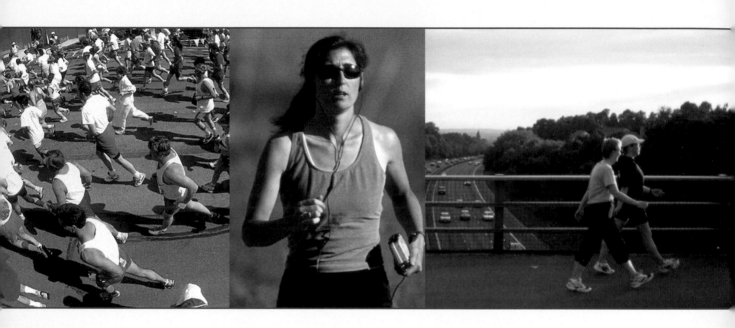

# BE **INSPIRED**

*How to take your walking further whether alone or with others, as well as an introduction to specific environments and the precautions they require.*

3

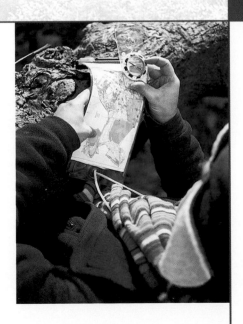

# WALKING **ON YOUR OWN**

*Surveys have shown that at least half of all walkers prefer to walk alone. Whether you spend the time listening to your personal stereo or simply appreciate a bit of "time out," walking alone need never be dull.*

The great advantage of solo walking is that you walk at your own pace and in your "comfort zone" without being "pushed" or having to walk at a slower pace. Walking with a friend can be a good motivator, but being tied to another's timetable means that you may not walk as frequently as you would like. Always follow the safety guidelines on page 94 if you're walking on your own, especially in an isolated area.

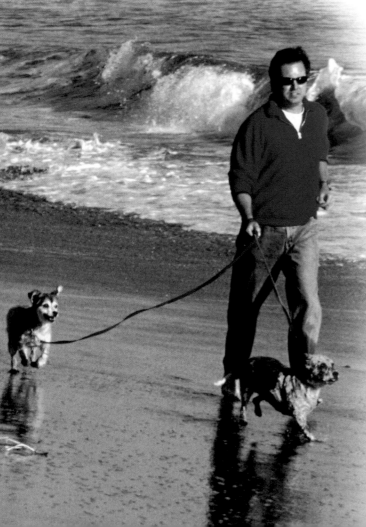

### Occupy your time

Although your time alone may pass quickly, you might sometimes feel that you need a bit of extra stimulus and encouragement. There are a number of ways you can use your walking time to greater advantage.

### *Boosting your memory*

While out for a walk, exercise your memory by recalling the names of streets or stores before you get to them, or by bringing to mind the birthdays or phone numbers of friends and family. If you're studying for tests, use the "method of loci" technique to help you learn. This involves taking each fact, word or date you need to remember and associating it with landmarks on your route. To recall the items, simply retrace the walk in your mind.

### *Meditative walking*

In traditional meditation methods, such as those used in yoga classes, you generally remain in a quiet room and hold one position, while focusing on an image, a mantra—a word or phrase that you mentally repeat— or the pattern of your breathing. Meditative walking works in much the same way, but you reach a state of calm by using your active body as your focal point.

### Take a dog along
*Studies have shown that being in the company of animals can greatly reduce stress levels. They also make good walking companions.*

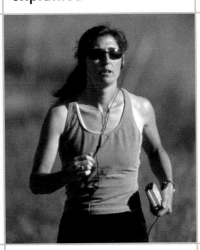

## WALKING TAPES | explained

Walking tapes and CDs are designed to help your pace. They are made up of music of a different number of beats per minute (bpm) to suit your pace. Tapes for beginners average 120 bpm, while intermediate tapes are about 135 bpm and advanced are about 155 bpm. Some contain tempo changes for the warm-ups, cool-downs and other phases of your walks. An alternative to ready-made tapes and CDs is to create your own. Simply count the number of beats in a song over 15 seconds and multiply it by four to get the bpm. Billy Ocean, "When the Going Gets Tough," for example and Madonna, "Like a Virgin" are about 120 bpm; while Elton John, "Crocodile Rock" is about 160 bpm.

To walk meditatively, use the following techniques:

■ **Find a route** Choose a place where you can walk quietly and safely for 10 minutes, such as a park or woods, ideally with some water nearby. Walk slowly but at a normal pace.

■ **Consider your body** Take each body part in turn, from your feet, ankles and calves up through your hips, belly and spine, and become aware of the movement of your joints and how your body parts work together.

■ **Relax and let go** Concentrate on contracting and releasing your muscles. If any are stiff, relax into your walk and release tension. If other thoughts enter your head, acknowledge them, then resume concentration. Become immersed in the sensations of your body.

■ **Slow down to a stop** As the end of your walk draws near, come to a gradual stop. Use your stretching period to ease yourself back to full awareness.

### EXERCISE YOUR BRAIN

Research has shown that people who take part in an aerobic exercise, such as walking, consistently perform better at mental agility tests than those who are more sedentary. This is because walking increases blood flow, which increases the supply of oxygen to the brain, keeping it alert and helping delay the natural aging of brain cells.

You may find that walking like this takes some getting used to. Try to repeat your walks a few times each week. Begin with periods of 5 to 10 minutes and gradually build up to around 20 minutes. As you become accustomed to such meditation, your mind will clear and you'll feel wonderfully relaxed.

### Walking to music

Music can be a great way to block out the world and, coupled with the aerobic activity of walking, it can help you relax. Mellow, instrumental music can have a calming effect, and upbeat tunes help you find a good walking rhythm. You also can buy special tapes and CDs for walkers, for example, with selections that help you maintain your pace (see box, above).

If you listen to music while you walk, make sure you're not so absorbed that you fail to notice what is going on around you. It's easy to underestimate how much you rely on your hearing when crossing roads and you need to be aware in case people come up behind you. Using one earphone only can be a good solution.

# WALKING **WITH OTHERS**

*Humans are social creatures. Strength and comfort is one thing we get from others when we walk together, but there are other benefits to group walking, particularly if the walks are well planned.*

At some point in our lives, most of us have started on an exercise program full of promise and enthusiasm, but after a few weeks have found it difficult to keep up, and have then given up on it altogether. One of the biggest obstacles to regular exercise is our lack of motivation. Walking with others can provide the incentive to keep going.

Joining a group is like getting a personal trainer at the gym. You are offered encouragement, provided guidance on technique, have your personal safety checked and are given new ideas. But a walking group can do much more than that. It won't cost you anything and you can meet a raft of new friends.

There is strong evidence that the nearer to home the walking group, the more likely you are to attend. So if you want to join one, look for a group close to you. Search your local library, newspapers and the Internet for contact details. If there isn't a group already, you might want to start one up (see page 62).

## Power from people

Many people find that they exercise better and push themselves farther when they are with others. Most groups include walkers of all abilities, which means that you should never feel left out; there will always be somebody around to encourage and inspire you, if ever you begin to flag. Being part of such a group gives you the incentive also to attend walks regularly, particularly if they are at a set time each week. Not only that, but groups also can expand the scope of your walks, taking you to new places—whether it's in the city, remote countryside or even on trips abroad.

## Safety in numbers

In a recent survey, more than 70 percent of the women questioned said they felt vulnerable when walking alone. Safety has become one of the main incentives for people to join and develop groups. Walking with others gives you the confidence and companionship to

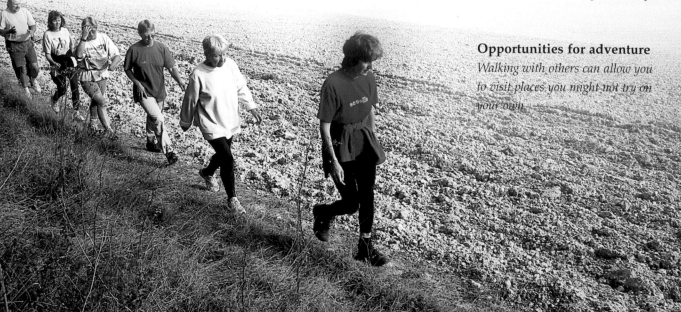

**Opportunities for adventure**
*Walking with others can allow you to visit places you might not try on your own.*

go out and walk when and where you want. Group walking also can help ensure that you don't put yourself at risk; there is always someone around to give you advice on your technique and check that you're working at a good level without overdoing it. Group leaders are usually trained in first aid, so if there is an injury, it's reassuring to know someone is on hand to offer treatment.

## The friendship factor

Family and work-related responsibilities often mean there is little opportunity to forge new friendships locally. A walking group makes available immediately a reliable and supportive community. Your social life is bound to gain, as you meet like-minded individuals who can become friends for life. In fact, you may find walking with others so enjoyable that you forget you're exercising and that your body is benefiting.

## Charity walks

If you're already reasonably fit and a fairly regular walker, why not give your walking a purpose and walk for a cause. Charity walks are a great way of getting involved in your community and can do tremendous good for an organization, both through the money they raise and the awareness they create. Participants number 20 to 20,000; events range from 2 to 3 miles (3 to 5 km) around your local parks to long hikes on national trails. They can even take you to such exotic locations as the Atlas Mountains of North Africa or the glaciers of Iceland.

Nearly all the big charitable organizations run annual "walkathons." Find out what's around by contacting them directly, or by looking on community bulletin boards or in newspapers. Alternatively, you could keep it local and organize a walk yourself, perhaps raising money for your neighborhood school or hospital. Try to raise sponsors as far in advance as possible. Supplement what you raise through friends, family and neighbors by getting your workplace or a local company to sponsor you.

*Walkers' tips*

## GETTING INVOLVED

### Go on a walking vacation
*This is a great way to get to know people with similar interests and aims and to experience new landscapes and cultures.*

### Visit the mall
*Walking among busy shoppers is great if you don't want to get involved in a group but want the benefits of communal walking.*

### Get a group together
*If you know what you want from walking you may gain satisfaction from getting similar individuals to join you.*

### Walk for charity
*Working for a cause alongside others gives you a sense of purpose.*

### Join an association
*If you're interested in a particular type of walking, such as racewalking or orienteering, contact a national association to find out about groups in your area.*

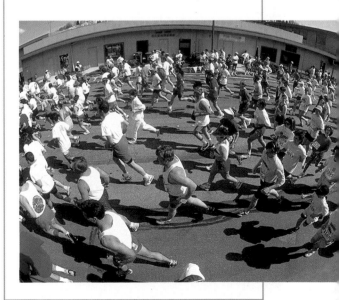

## How to set up a walking group

It can be an extremely rewarding experience to organize like-minded individuals to walk together. Not only is it a chance for you to help increase the physical and mental well-being of everyone involved, but walking groups can even save lives. If you encourage 60 to 70 healthy, but inactive, middle-aged people to take up walking, then each year you'll have prevented one of them from having a stroke or heart attack. Helping to achieve such a positive benefit is immensely satisfying, and so, too, is the happiness, confidence and sense of relaxation that good company provides.

This section gives you some advice about forming a walking group. For information on organizing walks and planning schedules, see pages 174 to 177.

### Do your research

You may have looked for walking groups in your area already, but found they don't offer quite what you want. If this is the case, then why not form your own group? If you're relatively new to walking, you can aim your group at other beginners, covering short distances in the local area. If you decide to go for it, existing hiking or racewalk groups can be a help, providing you with contacts and advice on all sorts of issues. If you stay in touch with them, they may also be able to refer potential members to you and vice versa.

National organizations are another great source of information on issues such as training and insurance. Search your local library, newspapers or the Internet for contact details. Some national walking organizations may have branches in your area already or might consider setting one up. It can be easier to establish a group with this level of backing. Refer to the Resources section for contact information (see pages 184 to 187).

### Safety first

If you're regularly in charge of group walks, you need to consider taking out a good insurance policy. Walking organizations may be able to advise you on the best companies to contact or provide you with insurance themselves. Insurers will often have minimum standards and requirements that must be met before

---

*Walkers' tips*

## GROUP ETIQUETTE

### Understand the goals
*Make sure that you know what's expected of you, the distance and duration of the walk, for example—and that you're happy to partake.*

### Stay together
*Wait for the back of the group to catch up, unless instructed otherwise. Then allow these walkers time to catch their breath.*

### Look out for each other
*If a group member starts to feel ill or is injured, at least one of the group must stay behind while others go for help.*

### Be considerate
*Chat as you walk, but be aware that others may prefer silence. An advantage of a big group is that you usually find like-minded people to suit your mood.*

### Ask ahead before taking your dog
*Make sure you take your dog only if it does not annoy others. Some people might not want a dog's company, in which case, consider setting up or joining a dog walkers' group.*

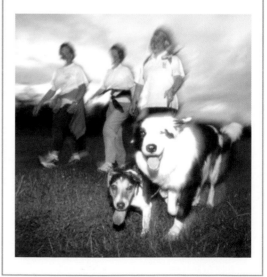

## ROUTE PLANNING | explained

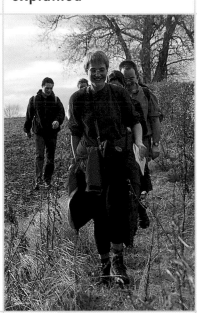

If you're setting up a walking group, you'll need to plan appropriate routes that correspond to the group's level. Designing a walk can be almost an artistic composition as you introduce buildings, neighborhoods, parks, fields, and woods to create a varied and balanced route. A point of focus for a walk, such as a church or a park, provides a destination as well as an identity. Setting off with spacious views can be energizing; in contrast, ending a walk with open views can be demoralizing and make your goal look far away. Tackle hills toward the middle of the walk, after walkers have warmed up but before they're tired. Try out the walk before you set it for others so you can tell them how long it will take and about any features along the way or about minor hazards, such as broken paving slabs. Check a circular route and then go the other direction. It's surprising how a walk can come together by just turning it around.

you're fully covered. You may, for example, need to supply filled out health questionnaires on participants and have at least two qualified first aiders on all walks.

As a walk leader or organizer, you're responsible for the health and safety of your group members. Each new walker should fill out a health questionnaire (like the one on page 97). This identifies anyone with a health problem who may need medical advice before increasing activity, and also makes you aware of the level at which each person should exercise. You must be trained in basic first aid, including CPR (see box, page 116), and should always carry a cell phone. Good map reading skills are another essential. If someone is injured or sick, you must be prepared to stay with the person and send two others for help.

### Active recruitment

You can start a walking group just among friends and family. However, the more people are involved, the more fun and productive your group can be, with people walking at different times throughout the week and a greater range of ages and abilities. Consider holding a public meeting at a community center to gauge the level of interest and find out the times people are available. You may be able to recruit fellow leaders, too. Ask a local health professional to discuss the benefits of walking and endorse your scheme.

Advertise in public places that might attract potential walkers, such as in the local newspaper, doctors' offices, community bulletin boards, malls, drugstores and local gyms. Give a telephone number or e-mail address so that people can contact you with questions and so that you can ascertain how many people are interested.

### Goals and expectations

One major advantage of walking in a group is that you can share your enthusiasm with people of similar interests, but you need to consider what other group members want from their walks. If you're racewalking (see page 86), you all need to be of similar fitness levels and walk at a fast pace. On the other hand, if you're organizing groups for beginners make this clear from the start so that nobody is disappointed. If you are part of a group, make sure you act responsibly and with courtesy (see box, opposite).

## Contrasting locations

A walking vacation can take you to landscapes that you'd never get to see from inside a car or a tour bus. Deserts, alpine ranges, gorges, canyons and coastlines all provide exciting walking environments. A trek to a famous ruin or monument can help you learn about the history and culture of the country, too. Some well-known walking routes include: The Inca Trail in Peru to the famous lost city of Machu Picchu, the Great Wall of China, and the Conquerors' Route in Mexico, which runs through steep canyons, green valleys, tropical rain forest and hot springs.

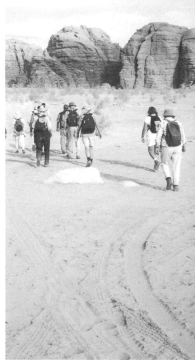
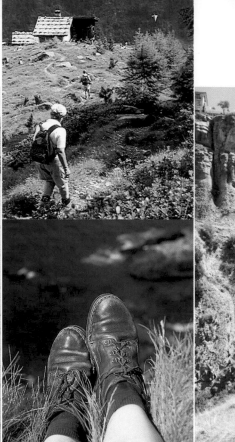

## Preparing for a walking vacation

Organized walking trips are at the opposite end of the "If it's-Tuesday-we-must-be-in-Greece" type of tour. Instead of speeding through a number of countries, without really learning about any, you'll experience a country, or part of it, in depth—becoming familiar with both the countryside and cities, visiting landmarks, tasting the food and meeting the local people.

There are many different styles of vacation, so choose carefully. Some companies have detailed group itineraries, while others will take you to an area, provide information and let you plan walks yourself. Check, also, on the size of the group you'll be with.

Before you book a trip, check it doesn't require more preparation than you can manage. Be ambitious, but realistic. If you're an inexperienced walker, don't try crossing the Gobi desert in three weeks. You'll enjoy it much more if you aren't overextended. Walking on the lower slopes of the Alps might suit you better. Decide whether you want to be based in one place and explore an area thoroughly or walk a particular route

during the course of a trip. If you go for the second option, but don't fancy carrying your luggage, select a tour company that will pick up your bags each morning and drop them at your next scheduled hotel. Find out how many miles you'll be covering each day and the type of terrain, so you don't prepare for a 2-hour-a-day walk on flat terrain only to face a 5-hour-a-day mountain hike. Use the programs in Chapter 6 to get in shape. A walking vacation should leave you feeling energized.

### Do your research

For a walking vacation, a little background knowledge goes a long way. Find out all you can about the weather in the region you'll visit—you can find a five-day weather forecast for almost anywhere in the world at www.metoffice.com. Learn all you can about the local culture, plants and wildlife. It shows respect to be able to greet local people in their language, and it's always appreciated. Your vacation experience can be enhanced if you can identify some native birds, mammals and plants, or understand the area's history.

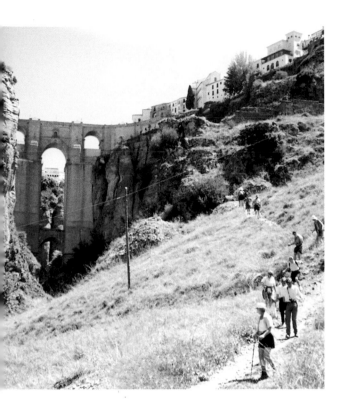

## ✓ WHAT DO I NEED?

❑ **Clothing** Wear lightweight, good-quality waterproof garments.

❑ **Footwear** Choose comfortable shoes and make sure you've tried them out before your vacation.

❑ **Basics** Never be without a water bottle, money, cell phone or camera.

❑ **Health essentials** Take malaria tablets, insect repellent, a basic first-aid kit and any prescription medication you need.

❑ **Information** Carry a pocket-sized map of the local area and a mini guidebook.

❑ **Protection** Take sunscreen with an SPF of at least 15 and wear a hat to protect from sun and wind.

### Vacation health

Make sure you've had the necessary vaccinations—don't leave them to the last minute, when there's not enough time for them to be effective. Malaria is on the increase globally. In North America, more than 1,400 people return from vacation each year to be diagnosed with malaria, largely because they failed to take malaria tablets or didn't take them for long enough. Make sure that you bring the correct number of tablets with you and that you know exactly when to take them.

If cholera is endemic in the regions you're visiting, make sure you wash all fruits, vegetables and salad, and use bottled water to drink or to brush your teeth. If you're uncertain about any of these health requirements, check with the Centers for Disease Control and Prevention, a great website for travelers' health at www.cdc.gov/travel/. Or in Canada, check with Health Canada at www.hc-sc.gc.ca. If you take regular medications, make sure you've packed enough, and have some in reserve. You may need a letter from your doctor to explain your prescription to customs officers, particularly if you need syringes. Remember to pack insect repellent—look for a product containing at least 40 percent DEET, the active ingredient that wards off bugs and mosquitoes.

### Perfect packing

The cardinal rule is: Don't bring too much. This is particularly true if you'll be carrying everything on your back. A camera, money, cell phone, small first-aid kit, water bottle and appropriate clothing are the essentials. Heavy books and large binoculars may lose their appeal halfway up the baking Sicilian hills.

The climate determines the type of clothing you'll take. Don't forget that 59°F (15°C) may feel cold while you're standing still, but you'll warm up fast as you walk, because of the body heat you generate. If you're walking in the mountains, carry lightweight, good-quality waterproof outerwear that can be carried when you're overheated but will keep you warm if it becomes cold and wet. If your walking boots are new, break them in for at least a month prior to your trip.

## Walking for pilgrimage

Throughout history, people have made pilgrimages to shrines or places that are sacred to them. For some this is a religious obligation, for others it's a time of personal discovery. It might be an opportunity to walk alone and concentrate on your inner thoughts, or an occasion to walk with others with a common purpose. Whatever the reason, the act of traveling can be as important as the destination itself.

The number of people going on pilgrimages increases each year. Traditionally, these routes are traveled on foot, and a journey might last weeks or months and include time for contemplation and prayer. In some places you'll be able to seek guidance from religious leaders. Many people choose a route associated with their particular religion, such as Muslim pilgrimages to Mecca, Catholic visits to Lourdes and Christian trips to the Holy Land. Pilgrimages can, however, be for more secular reasons, and many routes are simply fascinating and beautiful places to walk.

If you want to find out more about the walks on offer, check with your local church, community center or with specialist tour operators, many of which have Internet sites (see Resources, pages 184 to 187). Some companies offer special deals: for example, free travel for you if you organize and arrange travel for a group.

### Preparing for pilgrimage

Traditional routes can be hundreds of miles long, and, though you may not choose to walk the whole trail, you need to make sure that you're capable of reaching your personal goals. Consider the following:

- **Read up** At least three months before you go, buy as many maps and books on the route as you can.
- **Learn from others' experiences** Speak to people who have walked the route before. Pilgrims often post accounts of their journey on websites devoted to a particular route. With some of the more popular pilgrimages, you can even attend workshops to get tips and advice.

*"My father considered a walk among the mountains as the equivalent of churchgoing."*

ALDOUS HUXLEY

## PILGRIMAGES *for happiness*

► Having a goal for your walk can give you a great sense of purpose.

► If you need inspiration, where better to find it than on a route steeped in history and emotion.

► Following such trails brings clarity to many who feel they need a break from their everyday lives and time to think.

► A pilgrimage might take you to places you'd never dreamed of visiting and help you feel in harmony with the natural world.

► The knowledge that so many have traveled this same route can instill a sense of belonging, comfort and peace.

► There are sometimes retreats or religious places you can visit along the way to learn about meditation or spiritual pursuits.

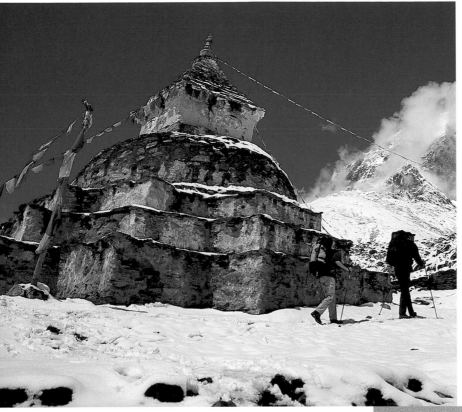

### The roof of the world

*Prayer flags flutter above a Buddhist stupa on the route to Mount Everest. Trekkers from across the world make the journey to Nepal, attracted by the imposing Hindu and Buddhist shrines and the pristine mountain scenery.*

### The Way of St. James

*This is a famous pilgrimage to the city of Santiago de Compostela in Northern Spain. The traditional route covers 500 miles (800 km) and takes a month to complete.*

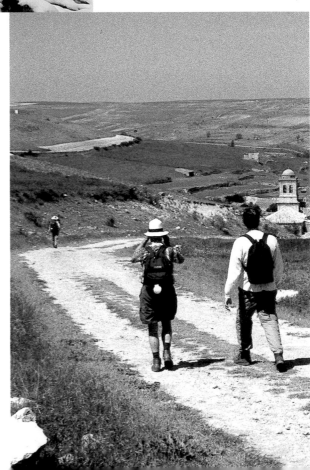

■ **Draw up a schedule** Once you have all the facts, draw up a timetable. Work out how many miles you can do in a day (see page 83) and don't forget to factor in rough terrain and points of interest, as these will all add to your time. Include rest days— you should take at least one day off a week.

■ **Get in shape** When you know how far you'll be walking each day, choose an appropriate training program. Use the Intermediate Program (see pages 152 to 153) to reach a good level of fitness and then gradually increase the duration of your walks each week. If six weeks into your training you find that this level is too much, you may need to alter your plans.

■ **Consider your accommodation** Many routes have ancient monasteries, retreats, hotels or inns along the way—you may have to book. Find out where you can get food and water; there may be stretches of the walk on which you have to carry your own.

# EXPLORING **NEW PLACES**

*It can be tempting to stick with a favorite local walk, but you may be missing out. This section gives you ideas for walks in different places and tips on how to remain comfortable and safe in various terrains and climates.*

Have you ever walked any local towpaths or river roads? Or heard about a trail in the mountains with a good inn nearby? There may be places in your own backyard which you may not know about. Why not pick up a map and see what's out there? If you do want to be more adventurous and tackle extreme environments, such as mountains or desert, why not give them a try—these can be exhilarating and fascinating places to walk. The key to walking them safely is preparation. For ambitious treks you'll need to

dress appropriately and have some background knowledge. Short local walks, on the other hand, require only minimal preparation.

## A walk in the city

If you're walking regularly, most of the walks you do will take place in the environment that's right outside your front door. For the majority of people, this will be a city. The good news about walking in the city is that you generally don't have to spend time planning a

---

*Walkers' tips*

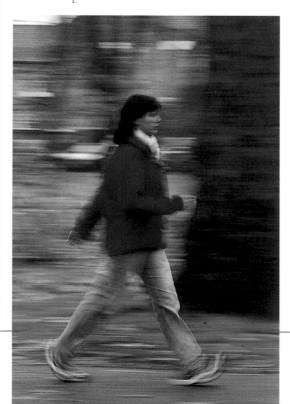

### CITYSCAPES

**Parks and playing fields**
*Parks often offer a variety of sights. Lakes, play areas, skating rinks, even zoos, while playing fields attract a lot of activity. In some areas, you can walk from park to park.*

**Rivers or streams**
*Many urban areas have streams or rivers flowing through the city center, and these often have paths running alongside them.*

**Golf courses and private land**
*Many golf-course owners allow perimeter walking, and landowners may allow public access to their land.*

**Suburban residential streets**
*These are quiet, well-lighted and often tree-lined.*

## POLLUTANTS | explained

Chemical waste products are present today almost everywhere. The main pollutants are: ozone, which occurs when traffic fumes react with UV light; nitrogen oxides ($NO_X$), emitted by vehicles and factories burning fuel; particulate matter (pollutants) from diesel engines; and sulfur dioxide ($SO_2$) from oil and coal burning. Lead from vehicle emissions plays a part, though levels have fallen considerably in recent years. Asthma sufferers are particularly at risk from pollutants (see page 102), but anyone can experience breathing difficulties if exposed to harmful levels. For those with bronchitis and emphysema, high pollution levels can cause breathing difficulties. However, pollution levels will rarely be so high as to make your healthy walk an unhealthy one. Be sure to check local weather forecasts. You may also check air-quality forecasts with your government agencies. In the United States, log onto the Environmental Protection Agency's website (www.epa.gov/airnow). In Canada, go to Environment Canada (www.ec.gc.ca).

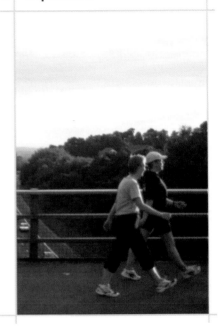

**Shopping malls**

*These areas are well-lighted and are particularly appropriate if you're concerned about safety or when the weather is poor.*

**Disused railways and other trails**

*Many abandoned railway lines have been converted to pathways. These are great places to walk, generally have even surfaces and can extend for miles.*

**Historical walks**

*These are great for a new perspective on your home town or a city you're visiting. Informative and entertaining guides can bring a place to life, as you learn about the city's origins, growth and development. Check out a local listings magazine or tourist office for walks available near you.*

route or driving to reach a suitable destination. Most of the time you can just get out there and walk with no more than a cell phone, some change, perhaps a water bottle, and the appropriate clothes for the present weather conditions.

### Safe in the city

There are certain considerations when walking in the city, but nothing that can't be solved with a few sensible precautions.

Try to stay away from heavy traffic areas and stick to pedestrian walkways and park areas. This will give you a break from noise and pollution. Wear brightly colored, reflective clothing so motorists can see you, and resist the attempt to "chance it" when crossing busy roads (see page 94). Most urban areas have some spots that are not particularly safe. You probably know which these are already. If not, your community center or police department should be able to give you advice. Signs of drug use, like discarded syringes or piles of liquor bottles, are indications of places where you could encounter trouble. Stick to areas where people congregate and, if you feel uncomfortable, invite a friend or walk with your dog.

### Timing is everything

One of the most important things to remember about walking in the city is that, as a walker, you're just one of many people on the street. You need to be sensitive to commuters, shoppers, cars, buses and delivery vehicles, and to the demands that these different groups make on the city. Think carefully about the timing of your walk and avoid the rush hours. There's no point battling your way through crowds. Not only will you become frustrated and stressed, but your walking technique will suffer because you'll be unable to get into a good rhythm and maintain good posture. If you don't feel comfortable in some areas after dark, an early-morning walk, when the streets are almost empty and the city is slowly coming to life, is ideal.

### Choose your route

You may live in an area where the main thoroughfares are always busy, even early in the morning. If so, you'll need to use your imagination and work out some backstreet routes that avoid the traffic but are still convenient to walk straight from your home. Make sure the route is not too complicated. You want to be free to concentrate on the pace or technique of your walking, not constantly trying to remember which turn you're supposed to take. If you feel like a change from your immediate environment, take a bus ride or taxi out to a less familiar part of the city and walk the route back.

The city can present obstacles to the walker, but it's also an endlessly fascinating and exhilarating place to walk. One of the joys of being in the city is simply watching people go about their business. Why not plan your route around a stop at your favorite café, and spend a few minutes relaxing and observing life around you, before heading back home? Or plan your morning walk around running your errands, so combining necessity with pleasure.

## Mall walking

Visit any shopping mall early in the morning or after hours and the chances are you'll come across an army of walkers speeding past the stores, turning sharply at the end of each stretch and steaming back down the other side. Mall walkers chat, nod to people they don't know and generally seem to enjoy their walks as social occasions. In this sense, mall walking represents a type of walking where you're on your own but at the same time surrounded by fellow walkers.

Mall walking is a particularly attractive option for people who live in an urban environment and really don't have a suitable outdoor walking area within reach of their homes. The weather is never a problem and there is mall security on hand, as well as rest rooms and water fountains.

### All-weather walking

*For older people, malls provide ideal walking conditions—flat, level surfaces in a climate-controlled environment.*

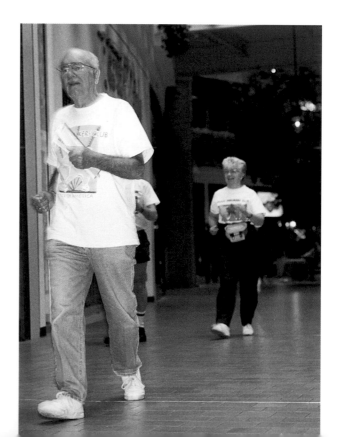

# MALL WALKING *for health*

▶ Flat walking surfaces and a climate-controlled environment mean you can still get your daily walk when it's cold and rainy outside.

▶ The distances are achievable for all ages and abilities, and there often are markers to spur you on and special programs to help you monitor your progress.

▶ Lots of facilities, such as water fountains, rest rooms, eating places, first-aid centers, make malls a convenient place to walk.

▶ Malls are ideal settings for those living in an urban environment who would have to travel a considerable distance to find a good outdoor walking area.

*"The longest journey begins with a single step, not with a turn of the ignition key."*

EDWARD ABBEY
Author of The Journey Home

## Getting started

Next time you're in the mall, try walking down one side, turning into each aisle, and then walking back along the other side. You'll be surprised at the distances you can cover. The pace is up to you. Why not try fast-walking the aisles, and walking the concourse at a more comfortable pace? Mall walking is great for beginners and older people—the walks can easily be divided into short sessions and there are benches at frequent intervals.

You don't need much special equipment or clothing to mall walk, as you'll be indoors most of the time. However, a water bottle is always useful, and, because you'll be walking on hard surfaces, you should invest in a pair of walking shoes with well-cushioned, flexible midsoles (see page 124).

The best time to mall walk is in the morning, before the stores are open to the public, or during office hours, when others are at work. Once the mall has been taken over by shoppers, you may find walking opportunities are more restricted. You might want to reward yourself with morning coffee with a friend in one of the mall coffee shops. You'll feel far more virtuous if you've spent the hour before your coffee striding up and down the mall, stoically resisting the temptations as the bakeries open their doors.

## Join the club

If you want to really get the most out of mall walking you should get involved in a mall-walking club. Call the mall near you or go to the information kiosk to find out if it has a club. If it doesn't, try setting one up yourself. The Internet is a good place to find mall websites (see Resources pages). Membership is usually free—the managers of malls are generally prepared to open the mall early to accommodate walkers, as they realize that walkers are potential customers who, after their walks, will be spending money in the stores.

Many mall-walking clubs devise special programs and produce maps of the mall with distance markers. Clubs also may provide health checkups and mileage rewards—often the walking club or program is sponsored by a local medical center. Store owners may provide discounts and giveaways for members, too. Some of the largest and best-organized clubs offer a whole host of services, such as free blood-pressure checks, low-cost or free cholesterol screenings, trips to other organized walking events and presentations and workshops by health and exercise experts, as well as many other perks.

If you're looking for a great way to keep in shape, meet other people and avoid the rain and cold, then mall walking could be the answer.

## A walk in the country

If you have access to rural areas, your walking can take you to places where you can soak up the tranquillity of the natural world, enjoy the sights and sounds of nature and experience the effects of the changing seasons. In an interaction known as "biophilia" (see page 19), our minds, released from the burdens of our hectic lives, open up to the subtle rhythms of nature.

### Where you can walk

The first thing you'll need to do when planning a country walk is check the accessibility of the area you wish to visit. Much land in North America is privately owned, so is not open to the public. Therefore it's best to stick to designated walking trails, most of which will be in national parks. For trails in your area, check with local hiking groups, park officials, or your Chamber of Commerce. Also check in bookstores, as many sell great books detailing walks in your area.

The national parks all have different types of terrain, wildlife, activities and rules. In some areas you may require a permit to walk the trails, and you'll almost certainly need one if you're camping. Check with the visitor center. Here you should also be able to get specific safety information for that area, such as weather conditions, treacherous sections and details of wildlife you might encounter (see below).

Most national parks provide detailed maps of trails. Walks may be graded according to their level of difficulty, typical categories being "easy," "moderate" and "strenuous." The grading tends to be based on the terrain, rather than the length of the trail. A route on smooth, level ground would be classified as "easy," whereas a "very strenuous" trail might involve some scrambling or easy climbs.

### Wildlife awareness

If you're lucky enough to see wildlife on your walk, admire it from a distance, but leave it well alone. We've all heard of the dangers of bears, mountain lions and snakes, but even seemingly harmless animals have their dangers. Squirrels might bite and even deer may charge in certain circumstances. Bites and scratches can cause infections, possibly even rabies, so don't attempt

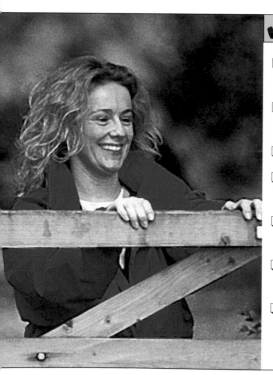

## ✔ HOW DO I CARE FOR THE COUNTRYSIDE?

☐ **Environment** Enjoy the outdoors, but respect those who live and work in it. Leave crops and machinery alone.

☐ **Access** Keep to public trails or access ways and shut all gates behind you—they are there for a reason.

☐ **Preservation** Leave wildlife, plants and trees in their natural habitats.

☐ **Pollution** Take your litter home with you and avoid making any unnecessary noise.

☐ **Fire** Guard against all risk of fire, and, if you're cooking or camping, avoid starting fires except in designated areas.

☐ **Animals** Avoid livestock and try not to disturb wild animals and their nests or dens. Keep dogs under close control.

☐ **Safety** Find out about any potential hazards on your walks and know how to deal with them.

to handle animals. Nor should you feed wild animals. It is not only against the law, but also it ruins their diets and can cause them to lose their fear of humans, as they associate us with food. Some animals such as bears can become a threat to humans, in which case they might need to be shot.

## Geared up for the country

If you're out on a country walk that lasts several hours, you need to be prepared for a change in the weather. If you're walking through an area of contrasting terrain, these weather changes can be magnified. Always check the forecast before you set off and take spare layers and waterproof clothing. Make sure, too, that you've got protection from irritating brambles, plants and insects. Pants, long-sleeved tops and boots that come above the ankle are ideal, and wear insect repellent containing DEET (see page 115). Gaiters (see page 129) will give you some protection, prevent you from splashing your pants with mud and stop dampness from soaking through your boots.

## A theme for your walk

Some national parks have themed walks you can join so why not combine a specific interest with your walk or get together a group of people who share your enthusiasms? Here are some ideas:

- **Birdwatching** Organized trails for spotting rare birds are common. Bring along a chart to record your findings and check against reference books when you get home.
- **Stargazing** Open areas away from city lights are perfect for studying the night sky. Take a star chart and binoculars. Sometimes amateur astronomers set up telescopes at certain points along the trail, particularly in mountainous regions.
- **Botany** Bring along a plant key and try to identify the species you see. Find out which plants are most common in the area, and then tick off the ones you find.

*Walkers' tips*

## IF LIGHTNING STRIKES

### Seek shelter
*You may have time to get to safety: Count the seconds between a flash of lightning and the clap of thunder and divide by five to estimate how many miles away the storm is.*

### Descend
*Leave high ground, it is more exposed.*

### Spread out
*If walking in a group, disperse so that if the worst happens, fewer of you will be struck.*

### Avoid tall features
*Don't stand near exposed trees, power lines, water towers or any other feature that projects above the ground. It is likely to be hit.*

### Get rid of conductors
*Keep metal objects, such as an umbrella, away from your body, and remember that some packs have metal frames.*

### Crouch down
*Make sure you're not the tallest object in the area by stooping, kneeling or laying down.*

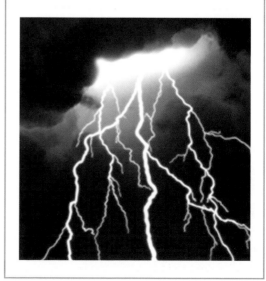

## Walking by water

Whether you're stimulated by the crashing waves of the ocean or calmed by the reflections of a lake, water can have a profound effect on your emotional well-being and provides a beautiful backdrop to any walk.

There are many different water environments, most of which provide excellent walking opportunities. You may not live near to the coast, but you're sure to be within reach of at least a stream, river or lake near which you can enjoy your walks. Check out a regional map or get information from your local library or tourist office on what's nearby.

### Exploring the coast

Whether you have sunshine, rain or an invigorating breeze, beaches can be wonderful places to visit, particularly at the start and end of the day when you may have them all to yourself. Walking on sand can be great for your legs; as it sinks beneath your feet, you have to work harder to lift your feet again, which not only helps tone your muscles, but also adds intensity to your walks (see also pages 46 to 47). On dry sand, however, this can be hard work if you're unfit and can be tough on your joints, so if you find it hard going, stick to the hard, wet sand near the waterline.

*"I hear lake water lapping with low sounds by the shore...I hear it in the deep heart's core."*

### W. B. YEATS

Alternatively, you could walk in shallow water to add intensity—water has 12 to 14 times the resistance of air. Stick to shallow water, no deeper than your thighs, so you can maintain your balance, and watch out for rocks and hidden ledges. As sand and water reflect sunlight, don't forget to wear sunscreen.

If you're on sand flats or rounding headlands, check the tides before you go (see box, below), as the sea can come in quickly and cut you off. If you're on or near cliffs, children will be eager to explore, so watch them near the edge and stop them venturing into caves. Avoid being under overhangs in case of rock fall.

### Tracing rivers

Trails that follow a river's course are well worth seeking out. Your surroundings can change dramatically with each bend. One moment you're walking by a huge

## TIDES explained

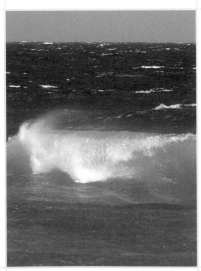

The alternating rise and fall in sea level is caused by the gravitational pull of the moon and, to a lesser extent, the sun. On the side of the earth facing the moon, where the gravitational pull is strongest, the ocean bulges toward the moon and creates a high tide. Meanwhile, on the other side of the earth, where the moon's attraction is weakest, waters bulge away from the moon, also giving a high tide. The rotation of the earth means that in most parts of the world there are two high tides every 24 hours, with two low tides in between. Working out the times of tides, however, is a complex operation. You can get tide information from local meteorology centers, newspapers or beach bulletin boards or on coast guard or national park websites.

industrial estuary, the next you're in a dappled retreat banked by trees. There is always plenty to see on a river walk, from the waterbirds and buzzing insects to people in sailboats and canoes.

If, for any reason, you go into the water or have to cross a river, do so extremely carefully. Even if the water is clear, depths can be extremely difficult to judge, because water refracts light, making the riverbed seem closer than it is. Read the box, right, for further advice.

Watch out for flash floods too. These are a danger in mountains and narrow gorges, and can follow just a few minutes or hours of excessive rain. They are also caused by the failure of a dam. The conditions to look out for are slow-moving thunderstorms or heavy rains from hurricanes and tropical storms. If you should get caught up in a flood, climb to high ground and avoid walking in flood water—even water that is 6 in. (15 cm) deep can sweep you off your feet. If you're planning a river walk in an unfamiliar area in a rainy season check to see if there are any warnings in place before you set off. The National Weather Service (www.nws.noaa.gov) gives daily flood warnings and flood stage information for the United States. In Canada, go to The Meteorological Service of Canada (www.msc-smc.ec.gc.ca).

## Discovering lakes

A lakeside walk is a perfect opportunity for relaxation, and following the circumference of a small lake makes a great route for a walk. If you plan on doing this, you need to make sure you can complete the route in good time and before daylight fails. If the lake is small, you'll probably be able to judge the distance by eye. For larger lakes, however, appearances can be deceptive. Check the distance in a guidebook, or measure it on a map, using a piece of string. Place the string against a

## CROSSING A RIVER ▶▶▶▶▶▶▶

If you have to cross a river, do so at the shallowest point and avoid fast currents. If you can step from rock to rock, do so carefully, testing their stability as you go. If you're in the water, cross slowly, letting your feet feel the way. Take a pole or stick to test the depth and help you balance. Always keep your boots on, or you risk injury from stones or glass. If you have a heavy pack, loosen the straps and be prepared to drop it if you fall.

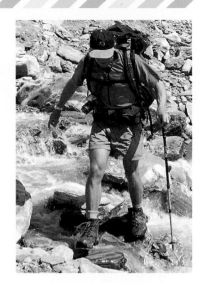

ruler length, before working out the distance using the scale. Take enough water and snacks in your pack to keep you going. Make sure you've got your cell phone too and some money, and tell someone where you'll be and roughly when you expect to be back.

It's never a good idea to walk across a frozen lake. You won't be able to judge the thickness of the ice accurately and it could very easily break. If you accidentally find yourself on ice, for example, if it is covered with snow, take off your pack and lie down to spread your weight. Shout for help and crawl to safety.

## SAFETY FIRST

If one of your group has fallen into the water, or you spot someone in distress, remember the rule: "Reach or throw, don't go!" Throw out a life preserver, branch or pole or make a human chain across the water. The important thing to remember is not to risk your own life trying to save someone else's. Never let yourself be pulled into the water by the distressed person. Shout for help, even if you think there's nobody around.

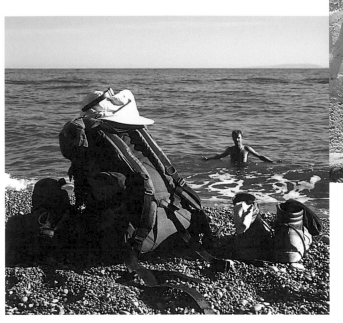

## Cooling off

*On a hot day, you can easily overheat when walking. Drink plenty and cool your body from the outside by going for a dip or wetting your head.*

## Walking in hot climates

Good weather and, if in summer, the longer evenings are great for walking. There is a sense of freedom when walking in lighter clothes and the warmth of the sun on your face can really lift the spirits. You do need to prepare, however, when walking in hot conditions.

### Be body aware

Listen to your body and you'll avoid pushing yourself too far. The most important thing to remember when you're walking in hot conditions is that you need to drink, drink and drink some more. The body's own cooling system works by secreting sweat through the skin. This evaporates as it hits the air and so cools the outside of the body. We have around 5 million sweat glands, which together can release up to 2 to 3 pt (1.2 to 1.8 l) of sweat an hour. These fluids need to be replaced to avoid overheating and the onset of heat exhaustion or even heatstroke (see pages 116 to 117). According to the American College of Sports Medicine, you should drink at least a pint (600 ml) of water before you start and after you finish exercise, and then as much as feels comfortable every 15 to 20 minutes during your walk. If you are walking for over an hour, consider sports drinks to replace sodium lost through sweat (see pages 92 to 93).

The extra sweat you produce in hot weather can make your clothes uncomfortable. You can, however, get clothes made from synthetic fibers that wick away sweat from your skin and help to keep you cool. Cotton garments are also cool in hot weather.

### Be weather aware

As well as being aware of your body, you need to be aware of the weather and how it can affect you. The perfect air temperature for your body is 66°F (18°C). Between 66°F (18°C) and 80°F (26°C) your body should be able to cool itself sufficiently. Above 80°F (26°C) your walking pace should fall to a gentle amble, preferably in the shade of trees. Make sure, too, that you take frequent stops to cool down.

The sun, of course, is the other thing you need to watch, as its ultraviolet (UV) rays burn your skin. UV rays are divided into three bands: UVA, UVB and UVC rays. While UVB rays have an immediate burning effect, UVA rays damage your skin slowly without you feeling the effects. UVA rays are, in fact, the main cause of skin cancer and wrinkles. Therefore, you should look out for sunscreens that filter out both of these rays. UVC rays won't harm you, as they're filtered out by the atmosphere. Apply sunscreen with a sun protection factor (SPF) of 15 or higher, which means you can stay in the sun 15 times longer than without protection. You can't always tell you're burning simply by looking at your skin: Press hard with your finger, and if the skin becomes very pale then red, it's likely that you're already burnt. Remember, too, that the sun does not have to be out for you to get burned—clouds filter only some of the rays. Reflective surfaces such as water, sand and snow reflect sunlight and increase your chances of damage from the sun. See page 114 for advice on treating sunburn.

The higher the humidity in the air, the more sweat you produce, because it doesn't evaporate off the skin to keep you cool. This is why hot, humid days can feel so uncomfortable. In these conditions, insects can also be more of a problem (see page 115). If the air temperature is hot and the humidity high—above 50 percent—you might want to save your walk for another day. If there is a cool breeze, however, this can help as moving air will increase the rate that sweat evaporates from your skin.

## ✔ HOW DO I COPE WITH HEAT?

❑ **Water or sports drinks** Drink a pint (600 ml) before you set out and when you return and then every 15 to 20 minutes during your walk.

❑ **Hat** Always wear a hat. Your head can absorb more heat than you realize, particularly between 11:00 A.M. and 3:00 P.M., when the sun is high.

❑ **Sunscreen** Use an SPF of 15 or above, and don't forget to apply it to your neck, the backs of your legs and the tips of your ears.

❑ **Sunglasses** Check that the lenses have UV protection, as the sun can damage eyes.

❑ **Reflective clothing** It's best to keep your skin covered when the UV index is high. Some garments have been treated to offer UV protection, and white fabrics are usually treated with brightening agents, which help reflect UV rays.

## THE UV INDEX

The strength of the sun is measured as the UV index. It is affected by the atmospheric conditions and where you live. Typical summer readings, for example, are: Chicago 5, New York 7, Dallas 9 and Miami 10. These figures can be found in most newspaper or TV weather forecasts. Bearing your skin-type in mind, use this table to check how long you can stay in the sun without protection at these levels.

| UV Index | Skin Type | | | |
|---|---|---|---|---|
| | White skin that burns easily, tends not to tan | White skin that tans easily | Olive skin | Black skin |
| 1 to 2 | ☼ | ☼ | ☼ | ☼ |
| 3 to 4 | ☼☼ | ☼ | ☼ | ☼ |
| 5 | ☼☼☼ | ☼☼ | ☼ | ☼ |
| 6 | ☼☼☼☼ | ☼☼ | ☼☼ | ☼ |
| 7 | ☼☼☼☼ | ☼☼☼ | ☼☼ | ☼☼ |
| 8 | ☼☼☼☼ | ☼☼☼ | ☼☼ | ☼☼ |
| 9 | ☼☼☼☼ | ☼☼☼ | ☼☼ | ☼☼ |
| 10 | ☼☼☼☼ | ☼☼☼ | ☼☼☼ | ☼☼ |

| Key | | |
|---|---|---|
| ☼ | Sun will not harm you |
| ☼☼ | Burn time of 1 to 2 hours |
| ☼☼☼ | Burn time of 30 to 60 minutes |
| ☼☼☼☼ | Severe burning in 20 to 30 minutes |

## Walking in cold climates

In winter it can be tempting to curl up in front of the fire, but we actually generate more warmth by keeping active. Walking is a great way of maintaining body temperature in cold conditions. At an air temperature of 32°F (0°C), a person who is dressed for the conditions but motionless will feel no warmer than somebody who is in an air temperature of 14°F (minus 10°C) and walking vigorously. Exercise can help keep you warm even when you're back at home, as it continues to improve your circulation.

### How heat is lost

The body needs to be kept at a temperature of 98.4°F (37°C) to function most efficiently. When the outside air is cool, your body loses heat as it radiates out through your skin and evaporates from your sweat and breath. The extremities of your body—such as your hands, feet and nose—are particularly vulnerable, because the body reacts to cold by rerouting blood supply from these areas to more important tissues and organs. Blood vessels in the skin shut down to prevent heat escaping. This constriction of the blood vessels can lead to the itchy, red swelling of chilblains, although walking should help protect you from this by improving your circulation. In extreme cases, the rerouting of blood can lead to frostbite—a condition in which the tissues of your extremities freeze. If your internal body temperature drops below 95°F (35°C), you are likely to develop hypothermia (see page 116).

### Keep warm from the inside

Your body has a number of systems for generating and retaining warmth, and you can do a great deal to help it. If you are planning a walk on a cold day, make sure that you eat enough carbohydrates (see page 90). The body converts food to energy in the form of heat, and it is necessary to have enough fuel for your muscles. Don't forget to drink plenty of water, too.

Muscle activity is essential for retaining warmth. It is either involuntary, in the form of shivering, or voluntary, in the form of movement. If you do start to shiver on a walk, however, it is not a good sign, as it indicates a serious drop in body temperature. If you've stopped for a rest, start walking again, as the activity will raise your body temperature. It's easy to forget, too, that once you've finished your walk and are chatting with your fellow walkers the body starts to cool quickly. Keep moving, put on more layers or seek shelter from the wind—moving air has a much greater cooling effect than still air, and this windchill factor can really bring the temperature down. Remember, too,

---

## LAYERING | explained

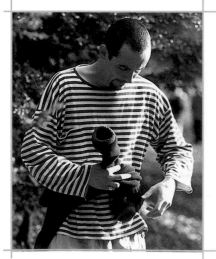

Dressing in several layers of clothing is the key to staying warm in cold conditions, and wearing two tops made of thin material will keep you much warmer than one thick layer. This is because the layers of materials trap air between them. This air heats up from the heat of your body and insulates you from the colder outside air. A windproof material, such as fleece, is ideal as an outer layer. If you get hot as you walk, layers are ideal, as you can remove them to cool down. Remember to put your outer clothes back on when you finish your walk or if you pause for any length of time, as the body can lose heat rapidly when motionless.

that you will need to warm up and cool down for longer on cold days, as the muscles, joints and tendons will take longer to get warm.

## Clothing for the cold

Wearing appropriate clothing is the most important factor in keeping the body warm. Always wear layers (see box, opposite) that you can remove easily if you get too hot and look out for the following when dressing for the cold:

- **Stay dry** Water conducts heat 26 times faster than air. In cold climates, therefore, you must stay dry if you want to stay warm. When clothes become wet they act like an enormous sponge, as all the air between the stitches of the fabric is replaced by water. This is why a breathable waterproof jacket is one of your best lines of defense against the cold. If you do get wet, change into dry clothes when you reach your house or car.
- **Choose synthetics** Many hi-tech fabrics will actually keep you warmer in wet conditions than natural fibers such as cotton. This is because they dry out quicker and tend to wick away sweat, which, if it stays on your skin, conducts more heat away from your body. Wool garments are good standbys, however. Look for fabrics with a tight weave to keep out as much of the wind as possible; fleece is ideal, as it is also lightweight.
- **Wear a hat** Half of your body heat is lost through the head, so wearing a hat is imperative.
- **Protect your extremities** Your nose and hands are the first to suffer in the cold. Wrap a scarf or a neck-warmer over your nose and wear warm gloves or, better still, mittens.
- **Warm your feet** Wear socks made with a loop stitch system (see page 127), as they trap air to retain heat, but also allow your feet to breathe.
- **Stay stable** Icy weather can be a hazard when walking. You can stop yourself from slipping by wearing cleats, which are like extra soles made of chain or rubber that slip over your shoes.

*"The exercising body is a furnace."*

## ROALD AMUNDSEN
*The first man to reach the South Pole*

### ✔ HOW DO I STAY WARM?

- ❑ **Clothing** Wear layers, as well as gloves, a hat and a scarf.
- ❑ **Shelter** Choose a route that's sheltered from the wind. Walk downwind when you start out and return against the wind once you've warmed up.
- ❑ **Dry clothes** Remember to keep your legs and feet dry as well as your top half, by wearing overpants and waterproof shoes.
- ❑ **Activity** Standing still for even a few minutes after your walk has finished will cause your body temperature to drop. Keep moving.
- ❑ **Food** Base your diet on carbohydrates, and bring a thermos containing a hot drink if you're likely to be out for more than 2 hours.

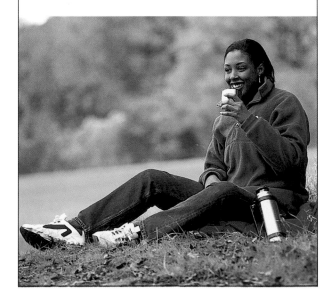

*Walkers' tips*

## COPING AT HIGH ALTITUDE

### Slowly, slowly
*Keep to a leisurely pace and listen to your body. The local guides on Mount Kilimanjaro say "pole, pole," meaning "slowly, slowly!"*

### Climb high, sleep low
*You can ascend higher than 1,000 ft (300 m) per day if you then descend to sleep at a lower altitude. Sleep no more than 1,000 ft (300 m) higher than you did the previous night.*

### Watch your health
*If you have symptoms of AMS (see box, opposite), do not ascend until they subside.*

### Stay well hydrated
*Make sure you drink at least 3 to 4 qt (3.5 to 4.5 l) of water a day.*

### Eat for energy
*Consume a lot of carbohydrates, as well as snacks such as raisins, nuts and energy bars.*

### Maximize your breathing
*Avoid alcohol and tobacco because they reduce your body's uptake of oxygen.*

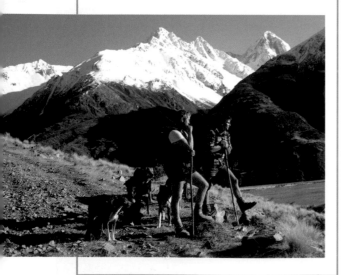

## Walking at altitude

The recent boom in adventure vacations to challenging locations has meant that the number of people likely to encounter low or high altitudes has increased considerably. Low altitude poses few problems for walkers and there are few low altitude areas in the world. In the few that there are, such as Death Valley or the Dead Sea in Israel, the main thing to watch out for is the heat, which is more intense below sea level. High altitudes, on the other hand, are more common and you may encounter them if you trek in the high mountain ranges of the world, such as the Andes or the Himalayas. These places can be incredibly exciting and exhilarating, as you experience the views and enjoy pushing yourself to new limits. However, it's essential that you prepare properly. Don't presume that a travel agent can provide you with all the information you need; do some background research yourself.

### Understanding altitude
High altitude usually means heights of more than 8,000 to 10,000 ft (2,500 to 3,000 m). At these altitudes you should watch out for rugged terrain, wind, cold, UV exposure, difficulty in obtaining clean water and problems associated with remote locations, such as the distance from medical facilities. But it's the thinness of the air at altitude that has particular risks.

Air at sea level contains about 20 percent oxygen. As you ascend from sea level, the air gets less dense, so that each breath you take contains fewer molecules of oxygen. At a height of 12,000 ft (3,700 m) there are about 40 percent fewer oxygen molecules in the air than at sea level. This means that you need to breathe almost twice as fast in order to get the same amount of oxygen into your bloodstream. When you're walking, your need for oxygen in the heart and muscles rises, so your breathing rate must rise considerably to meet the increased demand.

### Learn to acclimatize
Subtle changes occur in the body's metabolism to enable it to function with less oxygen. This process is called acclimatization. Given time, the body can

acclimatize to surprisingly high altitudes, which explains why entire populations can live quite comfortably at heights of 15,000 ft (4,500 m). If, however, you normally live at sea level and you go rapidly to the high regions of the world without acclimatizing, you may struggle. The rate at which your body adapts does not depend on your age, sex, race or level of fitness. Acclimatization is something that everyone must do when visiting such areas.

If you're walking at altitude, the key is to ascend gradually. Don't travel directly to high altitude. Start at below 10,000 ft (3,000 m) and rest a couple of days before setting out. If you do travel directly to altitude, don't do anything strenuous for at least 24 hours. Also, know your limits. At heights above 10,000 ft (3,000 m), limit your ascent to 1,000 ft (300 m) per day, and for every 3,000 ft (1,000 m) gained take one rest day.

### Build your muscular fitness

You can help your muscles adapt to the demanding terrain of mountains by focusing on hill walking in the weeks leading up to your vacation. Steep climbs work the big muscles at the front of your thighs (quadriceps) and in your buttocks, because you have to lift your legs higher than when walking on the flat terrain. Descents put strain on your knees and shins. Extra training will help you avoid muscle strain, soreness and shinsplints. Try to build up to at least 20 minutes of uphill walking a day in the week before your departure.

### Getting in gear

As long as you are sticking to trails and not visiting treacherous areas, you do not require too much specialist equipment to walk in the mountains. You should, however, watch what you wear. Good hiking boots with ankle support are a must, and you should always take spare waterproof layers with you. The weather can change quickly in the mountains. Sunscreen and sunglasses are essential, not only if you are walking near snow, which reflects light, but also because the effects of the sun's rays rise by 4 percent for every 1,000 ft (300 m) you climb. Poles can be useful to help you balance on steep descents.

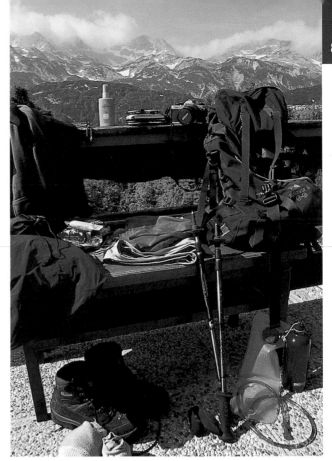

**Pack for the mountains**
*A large day pack is great for the extra layers, socks, sunscreen and snacks you need. A water pouch is essential for carrying all the water you need.*

### SAFETY FIRST

Up to 75 percent of those who travel to altitudes above 10,000 ft (3,000 m) suffer from Acute Mountain Sickness (AMS), with symptoms of: headache, dizziness, fatigue, shortness of breath or nausea. If your symptoms are mild, spending 24 hours at the same level may cause them to subside. If the symptoms do not go or become worse, then you should descend, as you could be at risk of more serious illness.

# TAKING IT **FARTHER**

*Once you've reached a good level of fitness, you may want to try different styles of walking. This section introduces you to the walking pastimes of hiking, orienteering, racewalking and marathons.*

The styles of walking described here present a fairly tough physical challenge and may require you to learn new techniques. These walks also bring great cardiovascular benefits but still without the risk of injury that is often associated with running.

## Hiking and backpacking

If you want to extend your walks, hiking and backpacking could be what you're looking for. Hiking involves fairly long walks that cover a variety of terrain and can last for a few hours or a day. Backpacking involves covering long distances, carrying all necessary equipment and traveling for a number of days at a time. Hiking and backpacking enable you to explore farther afield and to enjoy the benefits of being outdoors—viewing interesting scenery, discovering the wildlife, and escaping from your regular routine for a long period of time. Contact the American Hiking Society for information on organized hiking groups.

### Planning and preparation

If you've never hiked before, be realistic about your expectations. If you've completed the Intermediate Program on page 152, you'll probably enjoy a moderate day hike. If you're planning a longer hike over more challenging terrain, perhaps as part of an adventure vacation, you'll enjoy your experience more if you've trained beforehand. Aim to complete the Advanced Program on page 154, and choose a hike that allows an optional change of pace and route until you're confident of your abilities. Practice walking for at least an hour with your pack full. Is it comfortable and adjusted correctly? Do you really need everything in it?

Before you set off, make sure you're familiar with the route and that you've planned for all eventualities. Unless you're hiking with a guide, you'll need at least one good map of the area, in addition to any guidebooks. Make sure you can read the map properly and can take compass bearings in case you get lost (see

## Hiking equipment

You don't want to load your pack so heavily that it makes your hike a chore. Lightweight, waterproof clothing; sturdy, comfortable shoes; a basic first-aid kit; energy-giving snacks; plenty of water and a good map are the basics. Take a change of clothing and footwear for wet conditions.

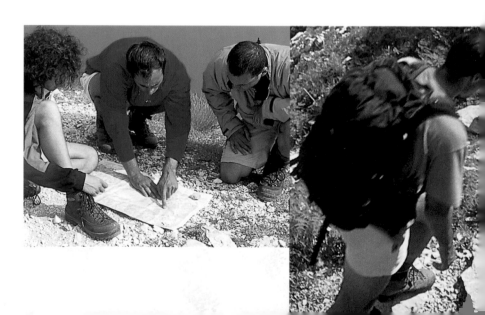

page 85). In particular, it's important that you understand contours. These are the brown lines on a map that join areas of equal height above sea level. When contours are tightly packed together this indicates an area of steeply rising ground, and as such, represents a particularly demanding phase of a walk. Also, make sure that you know what the various map symbols mean, can measure distances, and can work out how long a route will take you.

If you're new to hiking but walk regularly, you can expect to cover around 8 to 10 miles (13 to 16 km) in a day—less over tough terrain or in adverse weather conditions. Remember to factor in the time taken to walk to the trail head and for rest stops along the way. Plan to reach your destination at least an hour before dusk to allow for timing or route errors. If you plan to venture off an established route, leave your itinerary with someone who knows when you are due to return. If in doubt about the route or your map-reading skills, don't hike alone. Remember that cell phones may not work at certain points on your hike.

If there are Ranger stations on your route, call in for up-to-date information about the weather and your trail. Bear in mind you may need a permit to walk in certain areas. On most trails it's fine just to turn up but for some routes you'll need to complete a form at the trail head and there may be a fee.

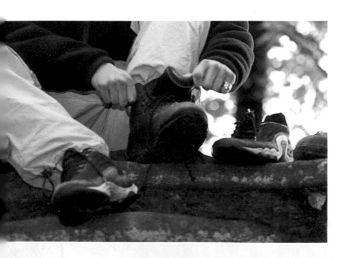

## ✔ WHAT GEAR DO I NEED?

❑ **Food**   Pack sandwiches, carbohydrate-rich snacks, and fruit. You will need more food than you usually eat, and extra in cold weather.

❑ **Water**   You need 3 to 4 qt (3.5 to 4.5 l) per day. Investigate the availability of water sources on your route, or take a water filter so you don't have to carry it all.

❑ **Clothing**   Take an extra waterproof layer.

❑ **Backpacking stove**   Fires are banned on some trails, so a portable stove is a must for cooking.

❑ **Emergency aids**   Carry a cell phone, army knife, first-aid kit and whistle—three blasts are recognized as an international call for help.

❑ **Orientation aids**   Take a compass and map, flashlight and a spare bulb.

❑ **Tent and sleeping bag**   Choose lightweight, waterproof items that fit snugly into your pack.

### Footwear and clothing

Because hikes are usually done off-road and on tough trails, you may want to consider hiking boots, which give more support and protection (particularly to your ankles and soles) over uneven terrain. Rigid leather hiking boots offer maximum stability but not much heel-to-toe flexibility (see pages 124 to 127 for more information). Make sure your boots are not too heavy—over just 1 mile (1.6 km) on level ground your legs will pick up and put down your boots about 2,500 times. When you know the terrain to be flat, and you're taking a short day hike, a lightweight boot or a trail shoe might be the best option.

Your clothing choices will depend on the weather and the duration of your hike. See pages 128 to 131 for more details. Always err on the side of caution and take an extra layer of clothing in case the weather changes.

## ORIENTEERING | explained

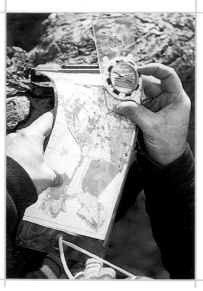

Orienteering has been described as "running while playing chess," because it's an intellectual as well as a physical challenge. Orienteering can be practiced on many types of terrain—in woods, parks, fields, deserts and even on skis in the mountains, and courses can be walked or run. It involves using a detailed map and compass to navigate your way around a course, with designated control points that are drawn on the map. In competitive orienteering, the point is to use the shortest time to find the control points in numerical order. Speed is by no means the only factor, since much of the skill lies in identifying the best route and finding the control markers. If you're looking for a way to take your walking a bit further, orienteering could be the right sport for you. The U.S. Orienteering Foundation and the Canadian Orienteering Federation are excellent sources of information, including ideas for juniors.

### Food and drink

Hiking requires a high calorie intake, and you'll need to eat and drink plenty to maintain your energy levels (see pages 90 to 93). If you're hiking for more than one day, plan your route via food stores so you do not have to carry everything you need. You'll need at least 3 qt (3.5 l) of water per day; more in hot weather. Consider taking a water pouch, which you'll be able to carry on your back and will hold more water than most bottles. Eat regularly or use sports drinks to maintain your salt and sugar levels—without food or these specially designed drinks, you could get muscle cramps.

If you're planning a long hike, and can't carry all the water you need, check the availability of water along your route. If in doubt, take water purification tablets or a portable water filter (see page 132).

### Overnight stays

On hikes that last longer than a day, you'll need to plan your accommodation stops carefully. In peak season, campsites and national park lodges book up well in advance, and you might not be allowed to stay in the backcountry; always check before you set off. Find out what facilities there are and if food is available. Most provide toilets and water and are a source of basic information about the area and weather conditions. The larger campsites and lodges are very comfortable, but tend to be expensive and must be booked in advance. Outside of the parks, shelters and official campsites are usually marked on maps. Measure the distances carefully and work out whether you'll be able to reach them comfortably by the evening. Most shelters are positioned about a day's hike apart but they can become crowded in popular seasons, so, again, check before you go.

Backcountry camping is usually prohibited because it can pose a threat to the local environment or because the area is surrounded by private property. Even where it's allowed you may find the terrain muddy or rocky. If in doubt, stick to designated campsites.

### Choosing a map

Even if you plan to follow an established route or hike with a guide or group, you should always carry a map with you, and learn how to use it before you go. Crossings might be washed away, or paths blocked, and you may need to find a new route. If an accident occurs, you may need to leave a group to find help. During rest stops, check the map to find your location so you feel confident about your position at all times.

This is also an excellent way to discover new walking routes for the future.

Maps come in different scales, with 1:24,000 and 1:62,500 being the most common. A 1:24,000 map means that one unit on the map equals 24,000 units on the ground. They also show this scale in terms of distance: for a 1:24,000 map, 1 mile = 2.64 in.

A small scale map is useful for planning a route, when you need an overview of the whole area. You'll be able to see features such as places of interest, water, tracks, major roads and contours. A large scale map will help you pinpoint your exact location when out on the hike, and is invaluable on a rural walk.

Outward bound stores sell maps covering the most popular hiking trails, but for detailed maps you may have to visit stores in the area concerned. Alternatively, you can buy maps online, including customized maps from specialist companies (see Resources page).

### Using a compass

If you cannot pinpoint your location or direction using landmarks, use a compass to take a bearing (see box, below). When using a compass you need to bear in mind the difference between true north and magnetic north. This is because your map works to true north (where the lines of longitude meet at the north pole) and your compass works to magnetic north. The difference between the two is called declination and it varies depending on where you are located in the world. On the east coast of the United States, for example, true north lies at about 20 degrees west of magnetic north, and on the west coast it lies at about 20 degrees east. Your map will tell you how many degrees from magnetic north a particular location is. Therefore, in order to establish your true bearing, you need to either add or subtract the bearing you get from your compass.

Luckily, many types of compass have built-in compensating devices to make this adjustment automatically, and it's certainly worth investing in one that has such a feature if you want to avoid the hassle of calculating the declination yourself. Otherwise, you could use the rhyme "declination east, compass least." In other words, the compass is showing the lower figure and you need to add to this to get your true direction of travel.

## USING A COMPASS ▷▷▷▷▷▷

Place the compass on your map with the base plate edge along your desired line of travel. Rotate the compass housing until the N of the orienting arrow points north on the map. Make sure the orienting lines are parallel with the map's longitude lines. Take the compass in your hand and turn your body until the red end of the magnetic needle is level with the red orienting arrow. The front of the compass is now pointing toward your desired destination.

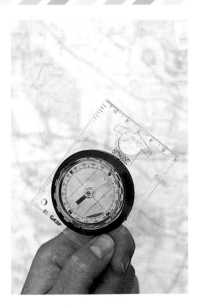

*"I want to be able to sleep in an open field, to travel west, to walk freely at night."*

SYLVIA PLATH

## Racewalking

Although walking has now overtaken running in popularity as a way to stay in shape, racewalking (sometimes also known as power walking), is still rather a minority sport, and one that receives little coverage in the media. It is, however, an activity that is growing in popularity, as more and more people look for demanding walking challenges.

The 50-kilometer (32-mile) racewalk is every bit as demanding as the running marathon. Perhaps one reason it does not attract the coverage it deserves is because racewalkers are often ridiculed for their rather odd-looking gait (see box, below). Racewalking is a challenging sport that takes hours of practice to perfect and years of training if you want to achieve top competitive speeds. Most good racewalkers can walk 1 mile (1.6 km) in less than 10 minutes, and 6 to 7 miles (9.5 to 11 km) in an hour. If you're the competitive type, or would like to take your walking to a higher level, consider joining a racewalking group.

## Marathon walking

If you're looking for the ultimate walking challenge, there is nothing more satisfying than successfully completing a marathon. Marathon walking is often done for charity, which makes it doubly rewarding.

Walking marathons either take place over the same standard 26.2-mile (42 km) course as a running marathon or over tailor-made courses of varying distances. It's becoming common for running marathons to offer a walkers' category—the Portland and Vancouver marathons are examples—and it's not unusual to see participants in the New York or London marathons walk the whole course. Often, shorter walking marathons of between 5k and 20k are organized alongside the full running marathon, over a course that is close to, but does not interfere with, the main marathon.

Preparation is all-important in a walking marathon. Even if you don't plan to complete the full course of a marathon, but are just walking a long distance for a

## RACEWALKING

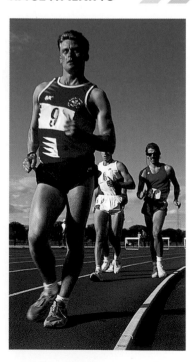

Racewalking is a succession of steps where there's no visible loss of contact with the ground. This means that your leading foot must make contact with the ground before your back foot lifts off, otherwise you're officially running. It's this fine line between running and walking that makes competitive racewalkers so prone to disqualification for "lifting." To racewalk successfully, you'll have to master the rotational hip movement, which is what propels your body forward. Although all walking involves some rotation of the pelvis of the forward leg, in racewalking this is exaggerated. By tilting the pelvis down and away from the weight-bearing leg, your center of mass is lowered. This reduces the normal vertical rising and falling of the body, which is counterproductive to forward progression. By flexing the pelvis forward, racewalkers also can place one foot almost directly in front of the other, as if walking on a straight line. This reduces any side-to-side sway, so making the gait more efficient. Racewalking places considerably more strain on the joints than ordinary fast walking (although has less risk of injury than running). If you can get the hip movement right, you should be able to racewalk, but check with your physician if you have hip or lower-back problems.

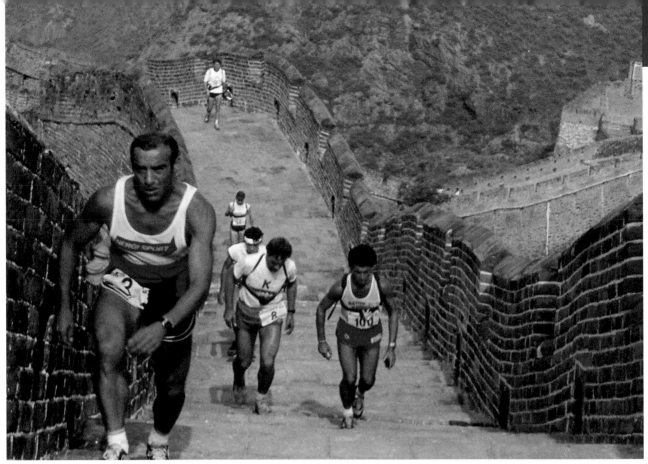

charity event, you need to put in some time and effort beforehand. You may be a regular at the gym, but this does not mean you're fully prepared. Walking works different muscles from those used for other physical activities, even running.

The basic training requirement for a long-distance walk is to gradually increase the distance of one of your weekly or twice-weekly walks. Given the demanding nature of this type of walking, you'll need to build rest days into your training schedule. Once you're able to walk at least 30 minutes on most days and a long walk of 90 minutes one day a week without pain or discomfort, then you're ready to start training. If you are starting from scratch and you currently do not walk at all, allow six weeks to build up to the 90 minutes, adding 15 minutes to the length of your walk every week. You'll need 15 to 18 weeks to prepare for a walking event. Try for three "hard" training days per week, including a 45- to 60-minute walk. Build in one longer walk of 2 hours in the first week. Increase this to 3 hours by the fifth week and 5 hours by week 14.

## Long-distance challenge

*The annual Great Wall Marathon attracts elite runners and racewalkers from around the world. Competitors have to climb 3,700 steps en route.*

### TYPICAL SEVEN-DAY TRAINING PROGRAM

The table below represents a good weekly training program in preparation for marathon walking. It's designed for someone who already walks at least 30 minutes a day.

| Day | Activity |
| --- | --- |
| 1 | 45-to-60-minute walk |
| 2 | 2-to-5-hour walk |
| 3 | rest |
| 4 | 45-to-60-minute walk |
| 5 | rest |
| 6 | 45-to-60-minute walk |
| 7 | rest |

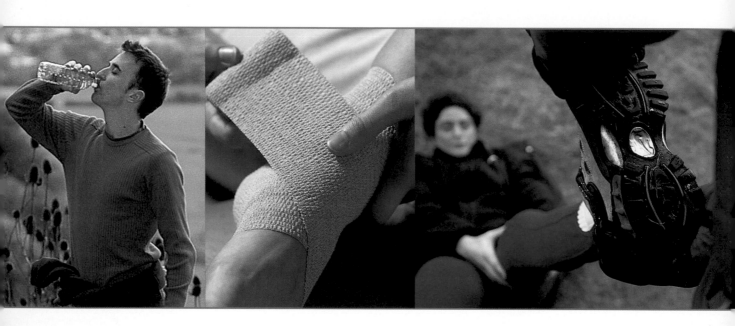

# HEALTH
# MATTERS

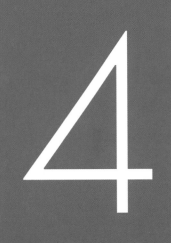

*What you can do to keep your body working in top condition. Plus, what you should look out for if you have specific health conditions.*

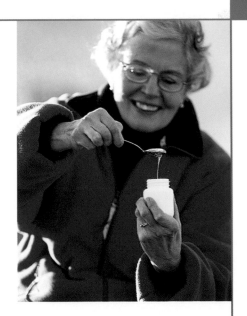

# EATING AND DRINKING

*Walking need not require big changes to your diet, as long as you eat enough food to keep you going and drink enough fluids to replace what you lose through exercise. This section tells you what to look out for.*

Taking up walking will certainly improve your health and well-being, but if you want to feel more fit overall and get the most out of your walks you should take a little time to consider the state of your diet.

## Eat for energy

Whether you're walking short distances or striding out for longer periods, you require energy in the form of food to enable your muscles to work. However, unless you are going on a walk lasting more than 2 or 3 hours, this doesn't mean you need to eat large amounts before you set out. Nor should you reach for any type of food for energy; some are much healthier energy providers than others. A daily diet based on carbohydrate-rich meals will provide you with enough energy for most of your walking.

### Healthy energy providers

Carbohydrates are essential if you want the energy you'll need for a challenging walk (see box, below). Basing your meals around good sources of carbohydrates and also keeping fat intake down will help you get the greatest health benefits from walking.

The best carbohydrates are natural sugars and starches, rather than refined sugars and starches (such as white bread, white rice and pasta, cookies, cakes and candy). The following are all great choices:

- **Natural sugars** Fresh and dried fruit and fruit juice, and some vegetables.
- **Natural starches** Whole-wheat bread and pasta, whole-grain cereals, brown rice, potatoes, peas, beans and other legumes, nuts, potatoes, bananas and some vegetables.

---

## CARBOHYDRATES explained

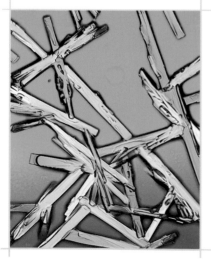

When carbohydrates are digested they are converted into glucose—a type of sugar that the body can use for fuel. Any excess glucose that the body doesn't use immediately is converted into glycogen, stored in your muscles and liver. Should your body require more fuel, this glycogen can be converted back into glucose. The slower the body releases this sugar, the more stable your energy levels. This is why unrefined carbohydrates are a better energy provider than refined versions—it takes the body longer to break them down. With refined carbohydrates, part of the breaking-down process has been carried out by the manufacturers—for example, when the husks of brown rice are removed to make white rice.

If your energy level seems to fall during your walks, this may be due to your meal patterns and the type of food you're eating. You probably need to increase the amount of carbohydrates in your diet. Increasing your intake of these foods also will add fiber to your diet, which will help your digestive system work more effectively and reduce the risk of colon cancer. Make sure that you increase your fiber intake gradually or you may experience abdominal pain, gas and bloating. It's vital to increase your fluid intake, too.

## Eating for weight-loss

Fueling your body with food is just as important if you're walking in an effort to control your weight—skimping on fuel intake will just make you feel lethargic and unable to exercise properly, and will cancel out any weight-loss benefits of your walk. Make changes to your diet by cutting down on fat and refined sugars and starches, and boost your intake of unrefined carbohydrates—as these release energy more slowly, they will make you feel less hungry. Choose fruits and granola bars for snacks, and, if you can't keep your mind off food, use your walk as a distraction.

## Preparing for your walks

If you're going for a day-long walk, you need to plan your menu around this. Start with a high-carbohydrate breakfast—whole-grain cereals and whole-grain bread are best—about 2 hours before you start your walk. As you walk, you'll probably need to refuel every 2 to 3 hours. Ideal sandwich choices include peanut butter, tuna or ham on whole-wheat bread, bagels or pita bread. Pack whole-grain muffins, fresh and dried fruit, pretzels, baked tortilla chips, granola low-fat bars or raw vegetables, like carrot sticks, for snacks. Drink water, fruit juice, vegetable juice or smoothies. Eating "little and often" (grazing) will provide your body with a constant source of energy for your working muscles and is perfect if you don't want to break up your journey for a formal meal. Grazing also can help control blood-sugar and cholesterol levels and boost your metabolism, which helps burn more calories. Always eat a meal or substantial snack within 2 hours of finishing your walk.

**Healthy sources of energy**
*When packing a lunch, make sure you include some natural carbohydrates to keep your energy levels high, without putting on weight.*

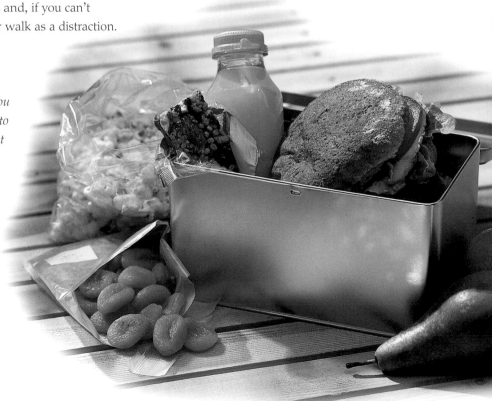

## Factoring in fluids

Water is essential to life and makes up 50 to 70 percent of your total body weight. Men's bodies, with their smaller stores of body fat, contain more fluid than women's. However, an adequate fluid intake is vital for both sexes to enable the body to function effectively. Water has many functions (see box, below), and when your body does not receive enough fluid to keep it working effectively, it starts to dehydrate. Symptoms of dehydration include: tiredness, dizziness, headaches and a general "low" feeling. If you've ever experienced any of these it may be time to focus on fluids.

### When should I drink?

Many people drink only when they're thirsty. This is not always the best method of monitoring fluid needs, because by the time you are thirsty, you're already on the way to dehydration. You can check whether you're drinking enough by looking at the quantity and color of your urine. If it's virtually colorless and there's plenty of it, you're taking in enough fluids. If it's yellow, or even darker in color, then it's time to drink. Your basic fluid need is about 2 qt (2.4 l) of water a day, equivalent to eight 8-fl oz (250-ml) glasses of water.

When you're exercising, however, you need more than this amount, because any form of activity increases your body's expulsion of fluid. Whenever your muscles work, whether on a Sunday afternoon stroll or a demanding day's hike through the countryside, they produce heat. This heat needs to be lost through perspiration to keep your body temperature regulated and prevent heat exhaustion (see page 116). The evaporation of sweat cools your skin, which, in turn, cools your blood and body. The more sweat you produce, the more you need to drink to replenish body fluids.

You should plan what, when and how much you're going to drink before you walk. If you're going only for a 10-to-20 minute walk, drink one or two glasses of water, juice or a sports drink before you go. If you're

> "All truly great thoughts are conceived by walking."
>
> FRIEDRICH NIETZSCHE

## WATER *for health*

▶ Drinking regularly helps your body eliminate waste and toxins and keeps your skin healthy and glowing.

▶ Your organs rely on an adequate supply of water to function properly, particularly the kidneys, where it helps prevent urinary tract infections, such as cystitis.

▶ Water is needed to produce digestive enzymes, which help you distribute all the essential vitamins, sugars and nutrients you get from your food around your body.

▶ Drinking is particularly important on a hot day, when it helps regulate your body temperature.

▶ Staying hydrated will make you feel more alert and energized.

▶ If you become dehydrated, you can get headaches; drinking water regularly can prevent this.

planning a longer walk, drink two or three glasses 2 hours before you set off, one or two glasses just before you go, and as much as feels comfortable every 15 to 20 minutes during your walk. Be cautious if it's hot and humid—this will increase your need for liquid, because the body doesn't cool off as efficiently in the heat and has to work harder to maintain its core temperature at 98.4°F (37°C).

## What should I drink?

Water is fine if you're going on a short walk of an hour or less; you're drinking simply to keep well hydrated rather than to provide your body with fuel. If you prefer the taste of milk, fruit juice or flavored water, then these are good alternatives. Of course, caffeinated and alcoholic drinks should be consumed in moderation, because the chemicals and additives they contain promote dehydration. If you choose to stop for a snack, make sure you drink liquids with your food. Also remember to check your urine color regularly.

## The sporting edge

You may also want to consider the sugar and salt levels of your drinks. On walks lasting more than an hour, isotonic sports drinks, which contain carbohydrates, can help you top up your fuel stores and give you a little extra energy. An 8-fl oz (250-ml) drink containing 50 to 80 calories of sugar can reduce tiredness and help your body retain fluid. If you're walking for 4 to 8 hours, then you should look for sports drinks containing sodium (salt), as exercise causes you to lose sodium through your sweat. Sports drinks are widely available, particularly in gyms and sports centers. Check the label to see how much sugar and salt they contain. Alternatively, you can make your own isotonic sports drink. Simply mix 1¾ pt (1 l) of pure fruit juice with 1¾ pt (1 l) of water. Then add ½ teaspoon (2.5 ml) of salt and stir.

*Walkers' tips*

## KEEPING HYDRATED

**Be prepared**
*Carry a bottle of water on walks lasting over 20 minutes.*

**Enjoy it**
*Choose a drink you like—all drinks count toward your fluid intake and are better than no drinks at all.*

**Anticipate**
*Drink before you are thirsty—thirst means you're probably already dehydrated.*

**Pace yourself**
*Drink in frequent, small bursts throughout your walk.*

**Be weather aware**
*Consume more fluid on hot and humid days, and avoid wearing heavy or unsuitable clothing, which will increase perspiration.*

**Refresh yourself**
*Keep drinks cool in a vacuum flask or by slipping a drink jacket on your bottle.*

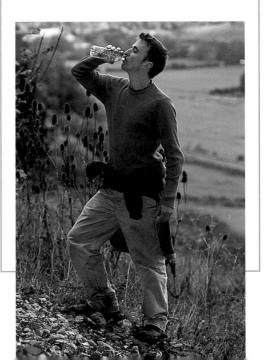

# PERSONAL **SAFETY**

*Whether you walk regularly in the city, suburbs or rural areas, you should take steps to safeguard your person and your possessions. This is particularly important when you're out walking after dusk.*

It's always best from a safety point of view to walk with a companion—this goes for men as well as women, who are just as much at risk of an attack. However, it's almost inevitable that you'll need to walk on your own sometimes. With a bit of thought and a realistic assessment of the risks, you can minimize the likelihood of an assault.

## Communicate

Always tell someone else where you're going. Let a family member, neighbor or friend know your proposed route and the approximate time you expect to be back. If there's no one home, leave a note or a message on the answering machine. Carry a cell phone with you in a day pack or fanny pack, and make sure it's charged. If you don't have a phone it's worth investing in one.

## ✔ ARE YOU PROTECTED?

- ❑ **Jewelry and money** Don't wear a lot of visible jewelry and take only spare change.

- ❑ **Whistle or alarm** Carry some form of attention-getting device and keep it in an accessible place.

- ❑ **Reflective clothing** If you're going out at night make sure you can be seen.

- ❑ **Get in training** Consider self-defense classes to boost your confidence and learn techniques.

- ❑ **Provide information** Let someone know where you are and carry ID and medical details with you.

## Dress wisely

If you're walking at dusk or later, or in foggy conditions, make sure you wear something white or an article of brightly colored clothing containing reflective material. Leave valuables and money at home, and don't wear too much jewelry—even if it's not valuable, it may look it. Avoid taking a personal stereo out at night; it is not only a target for thieves, but might also prevent you hearing traffic or people coming up behind you. Also, walk unencumbered whenever possible. In the rain, don't carry an umbrella but wear a waterproof anorak. Keep your possessions in a day pack so your arms and hands are free.

On the other hand, make sure you have some form of identification on you, and take along any special medical information, such as if you have an allergy to any medication, suffer from a condition such as epilepsy, or have to take a particular medication.

## Reconnoiter

Get to know your routes. This will do wonders for your confidence and feelings of security; unfamiliar areas can seem, and may be, threatening. Try to get to know new areas in the daylight, before you venture out at night. Take account of any obstacles, dangerous crossings or areas that are particularly secluded. Vary the time of day and the places you walk as much as possible so that you don't become a possible target. Don't walk alone at night in isolated areas. If you only have time to walk after dark, consider joining a group or walking in a mall (see pages 70 to 71). Try only to walk in brightly lit places, and avoid dark alleys, hedges, walls and unlighted areas. Be alert at all times.

## Self-defense for survival

Knowing how to take care of yourself in all situations is empowering. Consider joining a class that will teach you how to recognize dangerous situations and the basics of handling a would-be attacker, such as the defense technique, below.

Walk tall and with confidence; according to many self-defense experts, the less vulnerable you look, the less vulnerable you are. Avoid confrontations with other pedestrians, skaters or cyclists who might be in your way. Don't try and stare people down.

It's not advisable to carry any sort of weapon with you, because it could be used against you. Also, you might run the risk of being prosecuted for carrying or using an offensive weapon. You can, however, use

"reasonable force" to defend yourself. The best option is to carry a loud whistle or a rape alarm; this is often enough to scare off an attacker and should attract attention from passers-by. Make sure you have it easily accessible, as you don't want to be fumbling around and losing vital seconds. If you want to carry mace or a hot-pepper spray, make sure you know how to use it.

If you're threatened with any sort of weapon or if your possessions are taken, don't try to put up a fight. Make a mental note of your attacker's face, clothing and any distinguishing marks, including his or her voice and accent, and immediately report your reservations to the police.

## DEFENDING AGAINST ATTACK FROM BEHIND

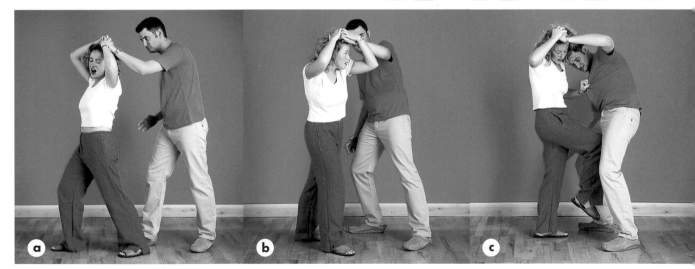

Should an attacker grab your hair, immediately scream and shout for help. Then plant your feet firmly, while you grab his hand with both of yours. Press hard down onto your head **a.**

While keeping a firm hold of his hand on your head, use the power of your legs to turn and face your attacker—this may knock him off balance **b.** Place your legs about shoulder-width apart, with your knees slightly bent for balance.

Now use your knees, feet or hands to defend yourself until you can escape. If your attacker's legs are apart, knee or punch him in the crotch area using as much force as you can **c.**

# BE BODY **AWARE**

*The decision to take up walking is an important one. If your goal is to be fit for life, this means that regular exercise should become an essential part of your life, no matter what your current state of health.*

Deciding to begin exercising is one of the most important steps you can take to improve your health. Walking can help you achieve greater fitness and well-being and avoid illness and disease. You'll feel the benefits of walking in both body—through improved flexibility, muscle strength and resistance to illness—and mind—through greater self-esteem and less anxiety.

Unlike many other types of exercise, walking is something that almost anyone can do, at any stage in their lives and whatever their state of health. There are only a small number of conditions and illnesses which would cause a doctor to advise you not to walk (see page 119), and, in fact, walking can be of great benefit to many other conditions. According to research conducted by the Cooper Institute for Aerobics Research, Dallas, Texas, people who accumulate 30 minutes of physical activity most days of the week cut their risk of premature death in half. This section explains exactly how walking can help with the specific conditions of heart disease, pregnancy, asthma, osteoporosis, osteoarthritis and diabetes, and advises you of any special considerations you might take when you're exercising.

## Think positive

If you have a medical problem, concentrate on the ways physical activity can bring relief from it, rather than using it as an excuse to remain inactive. The will to overcome an illness is often more powerful than the medicine used to treat it. A healthy mind is one of your best weapons in the fight against infection on the road to full recovery.

## Take it at your own pace

Your body has an amazing ability to fight disease, recover from injury and adapt to new environments and conditions, and it is always happiest when it's functioning between extremes of too much or too little. This is as true for walking as it is for any other activity. To get the best from your amazing body, you need to understand it properly and learn to respond to its needs. Don't punish your body with too much exercise, but don't neglect its needs through insufficient activity.

### MAINTAINING INDEPENDENCE

Recent research carried out at the University of California has found that the more active you are over the age of 65, the less likely you will be to lose your independence. A study involving 6,000 women over the age of 65 found that the more regular walking or stair-climbing the women did, the more likely they would remain alert, both mentally and physically. In the inactive group, 24 percent showed considerable deterioration of the brain, whereas only 17 percent of the active group had similar symptoms.

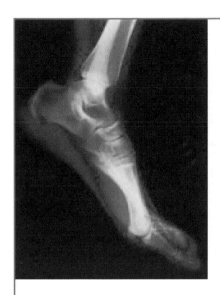

## Are you fit for walking?

If you are planning to take up exercise, then you need to know if you are physically ready. This questionnaire is designed to help you decide just that. Answer the questions below as honestly as you can. If you answer "yes" to any of them, you are probably able to take up walking, but must check with your doctor before you start. He or she will help you structure a safe and effective exercise program. If you answer "no" to them all, then you are ready to go; however, checking with your doctor before starting any new exercise program is always a sound idea.

❑ Has your doctor ever said that you've a heart condition, such as angina, myocarditis or atrial fibrillation—your heart is beating erratically—or have you ever experienced a stroke or blood clot?

❑ Do you ever experience pain in your chest or upper body when walking, or at any other time?

❑ In the past month, have you experienced any chest pain or upper-body pain when you were not physically active?

❑ Do you ever feel faint, lose your balance, become dizzy or lose consciousness?

❑ Do you have a bone or joint problem such as rheumatoid arthritis or tendinitis that would worsen when walking?

❑ Is your doctor currently prescribing any medication for high blood pressure or a heart condition?

❑ Have you had any surgery in the last three months?

❑ Do you suffer from epilepsy that is hard to control?

❑ Do you suffer from diabetes?

❑ Are you pregnant with twins or experiencing complications with your pregnancy (see box page 100)?

❑ Do you have an illness that is still being diagnosed?

❑ Do you suffer from any other medical condition, which you think may prevent you from walking?

## Walking with heart conditions

If you have high blood pressure, angina, or have had a heart attack or heart failure, heart surgery or atrial fibrillation—when the heart is out of rhythm—increased physical activity will be of benefit. Walking is the easiest, safest and most effective way of strengthening your heart.

### High blood pressure

According to the American Heart Association, about 25 percent of adults have high blood pressure (hypertension), and, of these, around 32 percent are unaware that they have it. As high blood pressure is a major risk factor for both heart attacks and stroke—a blockage or rupture of a blood vessel in the brain—it is important that you keep a check on it.

High blood pressure does not place any restrictions on your walking unless it's 200/110 or above (see box, below), at which level you should consult your doctor before undertaking activity. Regular walking will both lower blood pressure and prevent it rising.

### Angina

This is a chest pain caused when the coronary artery carrying blood to the heart muscle becomes narrow, reducing the oxygen to the heart. About 4 percent of men and 3 percent of women will have angina at some

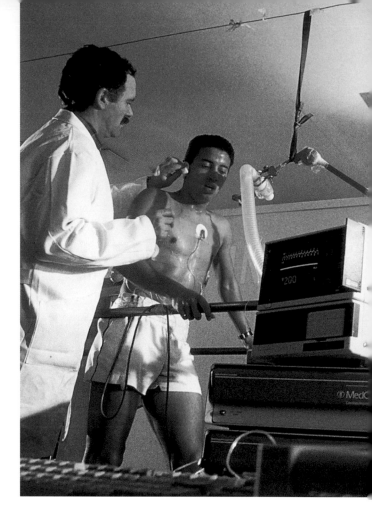

**Testing fitness**
*After a heart attack, fitness can be monitored while walking on a treadmill.*

---

**BLOOD PRESSURE** | **explained**

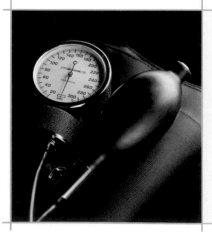

Blood pressure readings indicate the elasticity and health of your arteries. A reading will be given in two measures, for example 120/70. The first number is the systolic measure and refers to the maximum pressure exerted on the arteries, when the heart muscle contracts and the blood surges through them. The second number is the diastolic measure, and refers to the minimum pressure on the arteries, when the heart relaxes. If you have a high blood pressure of 150/95, for example, you can lower it to a more normal blood reading by exercising regularly and cutting down on salt.

point in their lives. Walking helps reduce your risk of angina by increasing the strength of the heart and allowing oxygen to be transferred to the muscle more easily. If you experience chest pain while walking, stop. If you've been treated for angina and have your medication with you, take it right away. The pain should fade and you'll be able to continue your walk, at a slightly slower pace. If the pain continues for more than 15 minutes or is accompanied by sweating or a fainting feeling, get medical assistance immediately.

## Heart attack

More than 1 million people a year suffer heart attacks. Most heart attacks are caused by a blockage of the coronary artery that supplies blood to the muscle of the heart. A section of muscle stops working and, although other parts of the muscle take over the work temporarily, it can eventually cause the heart to stop.

There are many things you can do to lower your risks of a heart attack, including cutting out smoking and lowering the amount of saturated fats and salt in your diet, but increasing the amount of exercise you do is one of your best protective measures. This is not only because it strengthens the muscle of your heart, but also because it increases the blood supply to your heart, relieves stress, lowers your blood pressure and cholesterol levels and reduces the body's ability to form the blood clots that can be the cause of a heart attack.

If you have suffered a heart attack, then walking can be a big step on your road to recovery. In the first few weeks following a heart attack, your cardiac rehabilitation (rehab) team will advise you on how much physical activity is right for you. Once you've been discharged, you can gently integrate walking into your routine and so reduce your risks of another attack.

You may find that you need a boost of confidence after your rehab program as both your mind and body recover from such a serious condition. Start slowly, walking for just 10 minutes a day, and increase your pace to a moderate pace during the following eight weeks. Remember not to overexert yourself and stop if you feel any of the symptoms in the box, top right. See pages 156 to 157 for a program to help your heart.

---

### ✔ WHAT ARE THE STOP SIGNS?

- ❑ **Pain or discomfort** This occurs in the chest or upper body, particularly the left arm.

- ❑ **Breathlessness** This will be uncontrollable and take a long time to subside.

- ❑ **Dizziness or nausea** This is a warning if it started during your walk.

- ❑ **Fainting** Watch out for this before or immediately after activity.

- ❑ **Palpitations** A fast or irregular heartbeat is a danger signal.

---

## Other coronary conditions

Atrial fibrillation is a common condition that causes the heart to be out of rhythm. Walking is an excellent activity to help improve the heart's irregular rhythm. Monitor your pulse rate as you walk using a heart-rate monitor (see page 144) or by regularly taking your pulse (see page 141). If you find your symptoms worsen when you walk or you are missing beats more often, then see your doctor.

After any major operation you'll need to be careful when it comes to exercise. Increase your activity slowly. Your cardiologist will advise you on the level of activity that is right for you.

*"The sum of the whole is this: Walk and be happy; Walk and be healthy. The best way to lengthen out our days is to walk steadily and with a purpose."*

**CHARLES DICKENS**

## Walking and pregnancy

Planning for and having a baby can be a confusing enough time without all the conflicting advice on what exercise is or isn't beneficial. Generally speaking, walking is an excellent activity before and during pregnancy, though, of course, the amount and intensity of walking you do will depend on the specific stage of your pregnancy.

### Prepregnancy fitness

If you are considering starting a family, then consider fitness at the same time. Building your health and stamina will not only prepare your body for the extra work it will need to do when there are two of you, but can also help boost your fertility. Walking can help you maintain a healthy weight and therefore a regular menstrual cycle and, by promoting relaxation and boosting your energy levels, it will also be great for your sex drive. Make sure your partner understands the importance of prepregnancy fitness too—regular walking will keep his weight at a healthy level and can improve his sperm count.

The greater your aerobic fitness, the less tired you'll feel when you become pregnant, a time when your body must support two beating hearts and two

**BOOSTING YOUR FERTILITY**

Research at the University of Adelaide in South Australia has found that overweight women who increase their exercise levels to lose weight significantly boost their fertility levels. The Queen Elizabeth Hospital at Repromed offers a regular lifestyle program called "Fertility Fitness" to improve overall fitness and give "your fertility a kick start." It has been running for nine years and has helped people optimize their diet and exercise prior to or instead of receiving fertility treatment.

circulatory systems, not to mention the extra weight you'll carry. Pregnancy, labor and the sleepless nights after delivery are times of immense physical and mental exertion. A high level of cardiovascular fitness will bring great benefits to you and your baby.

### Exercise during pregnancy

Most physical activities will benefit a pregnant woman; the only risks are from those sports that involve body contact or risk of falls. Check with your doctor on those you wish to perform. Walking is a great exercise for pregnancy, as it is relatively risk-free, and there are only a few situations in which your doctor may advise you not to walk (see box, left). Also, walking can help with specific conditions—it can reduce swelling of the ankles and lessens the pain of varicose veins, both of which can be made worse during this time.

Walking can bring benefits to the mind as well. This is a challenging time in your life, and there may be times when you'll feel overwhelmed. Escaping to a peaceful area where you can wander and think clearly can help you regain perspective.

### Listen to your body

It's important to be active, but you should also take into account your body's needs and changes. There will be times when you'll become very tired. Don't fight this. Allow yourself a rest when you need it. If you have to choose between a rest or a walk, just listen to what your body says. During pregnancy and for three months after the birth, you will also need to be careful of your posture when walking and stretching. This is because the hormone relaxin, which softens th-

**SAFETY FIRST**

Your care provider will tell you whether walking is advisable if your pregnancy is complicated by the following:

► Multiple births

► Bleeding, particularly after 16 weeks

► High blood pressure or considerable swelling of ankles and fingers

► A previous early delivery

► Development of the fetus is delayed

connective tissue in joints and muscles ready for the delivery, can make these areas more prone to injuries.

■ **First trimester (weeks 1 to 13)** This is the time you'll probably feel tired and have morning sickness. If you were fit before your pregnancy, then you'll reap the benefits now as your heart works harder to deliver blood to your growing placenta. However, it's not too late to start walking—it can't relieve nausea as such, but it can distract you from the symptoms. If you enjoyed more strenuous sports or physical challenges you may have to tone things down and turn to less demanding activities. Walking is ideal to keep you active during this time. Just don't push yourself too hard and become overtired.

■ **Second trimester (weeks 14 to 26)** With less nausea and tiredness occurring, you may find you can increase your level of activity. Many women safely continue to run and cycle during this time, so don't assume these activities will hurt the baby. If your fitness level was good before your pregnancy, then go for it.

■ **Third trimester (weeks 27 to 40)** This is when you may find the tiredness returns. Continue to walk regularly, but let your body dictate the pace and distance. You may become increasingly breathless during this period. This is from the baby pushing into the diaphragm and the increased levels of a hormone called progesterone. At this stage, it's important to wear properly fitting shoes, because the ligaments in the arch of the foot will be becoming less tight and less able to support you, due to the greater weight your feet are carrying. A shoe with a supportive arch is ideal. When you reach the early stages of labor, your care provider may advise you to walk around the hospital or at home to help the baby's head engage. It also gives you something to do.

## CALF RAISES

This exercise strengthens your calf muscles and helps improve the circulation in your legs. You'll find this particularly beneficial if you suffer from varicose veins. Stand facing a wall, about 2 ft (60 cm) away, with your feet slightly apart and knees soft. Keeping your spine straight, lean slightly forward and rest your hands gently on the wall. Look straight ahead, keeping your abdominals pulled in and your pelvis tilted **a.** With your weight evenly distributed slowly rise up onto your toes, lifting the arch of your foot as high as possible **b.** Check that your weight is forward and that your chest is lifted. Hold this position for a couple of seconds and then lower both heels gently, making sure they do not bang back down onto the floor. Start with 2 sets of 8 repetitions, and move on to 3 sets of 16 repetitions once you're comfortable with the exercise.

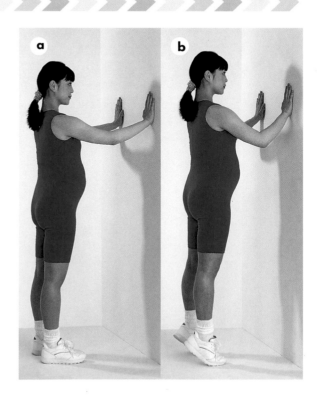

### Walking with asthma

Asthma is no barrier to being active; in fact, the more active you are, the more fit you become and the greater capacity your lungs will have to cope with your condition. If you are new to exercise, walking is an excellent place to start.

### Understanding asthma

This common condition is the result of the tiny breathing tubes or airways in the lungs becoming narrow so less air can get through. The linings of the tubes become inflamed and then swell, mucus (phlegm) clogs up the insides of the tubes, and the muscles around the tubes tighten.

Most asthma sufferers need to use both a preventer–inhaler and a reliever–inhaler. A preventer–inhaler reduces the swelling and mucus build-up in the breathing tubes and should be used every day. The most common preventer–inhalers are steroids and long-acting bronchodilator inhalers (such as salbutamol or salmeterol), which can be used from once in a while to two puffs, four times a day. A reliever–inhaler (such as salbutamol) is a "quick fix"

which reduces the tightening of the muscles around the breathing tubes, but doesn't reduce swelling or mucus build-up. It should be used for temporary relief from an attack. Asthma tablets (Leukotriene receptor antagonists) are a fairly recent development. If taken daily, they can prevent the onset of asthma symptoms.

Controversy abounds when it comes to alternative treatments, but almost everyone agrees that relaxation is good for your health, and walking an excellent way of relaxing both mind and body. The added benefits of walking such as warming the body, and improving the circulation, can also have a positive impact on asthma.

### A word of warning

Although walking is ideal for those with asthma, all kinds of exercise can make demands on your body. When walking briskly, you breathe in more air than when resting and it can be tempting to breathe through the mouth, bypassing the hairs in your nose that warm incoming air. This can result in coughing, wheezing, tightness of the chest and difficulty breathing as you get tired toward the end of your walk. To help avoid this, read the box below, and use your

### Walkers' tips

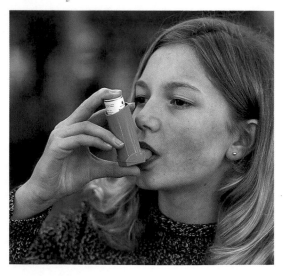

## PREVENTING ATTACKS

### Warm up well
*Ten minutes of gentle warm-up exercise helps build your breathing rate slowly.*

### Remember your inhaler
*If you have exercise-induced asthma then use your reliever-inhaler at least 30 minutes before you set out.*

### Check the weather
*Cold, dry days can aggravate asthma as it takes longer for your body to warm the air you inhale. Take it easy or wear a scarf (see above, opposite).*

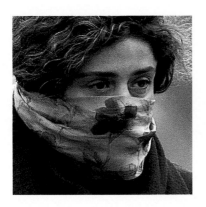

## WALKING IN THE WINTER ▶▶▶▶▶

The most troublesome weather for asthmatics is a cold, dry day. Usually, as air travels through your nose and into your lungs, it's warmed by the nose and body. But on a cold day, you may walk farther and breathe harder, often through your mouth, so the air doesn't have time to warm up. This causes your bronchial airways to constrict. Breathing through a non-fibrous scarf—for example, fleece or silk—or with your hand over your mouth can help. If you still have difficulty with your breathing, slow your pace and be prepared to use your inhaler.

reliever–inhaler at least half an hour before you set out and carry a reliever–inhaler with you. Don't skimp on the warm-up—it will help to increase your breathing rate slowly and is particularly important if the air is cold. Cooling down should not be overlooked either.

### The pollution factor

On the whole, air pollution is not as serious a problem for asthma sufferers as many people believe. The levels of many pollutants can actually be higher inside your home than outside. However, certain outdoor pollutants such as pollen, ozone (the main ingredient in smog), traffic fumes and microscopic particles produced by industry and diesel vehicles, can trigger symptoms and should be avoided where possible. Children are particularly vulnerable to high levels of ozone, especially when exercising.

When levels of these pollutants are high, such as near a road or during the summer, take care to modify your walking route and level of activity. Walk away from roads and fields where chemicals may be in use. Weather reports in newspapers, television programs and on websites will provide information about city pollution levels.

### Hay fever and asthma

If you are allergic to a type of pollen, use your inhaler and consider taking an antihistamine just before the pollen season to help build up your resistance. Pollen forecasts usually deal with the most common allergen, ragweed, but there are many others around at different times of the year, and you may notice a pattern developing in your own response throughout the spring and summer. Tree pollen occurs in the spring. Grass pollen occurs in northern latitudes during early summer. Weed pollen dominates for the rest of the summer and fungal spores peak in the autumn. The cycle starts again in spring. If hay fever makes your walking uncomfortable, investigate other places to walk such as in malls.

---

**Time your walk carefully**
*Pollution levels are at their lowest in the early morning or evening, outside of rush hours, so these are good times to go for a walk.*

**Breathe through your nose**
*Your nasal hairs warm up the air and make it easier to breathe.*

**Check the pollen count**
*If you also get hay fever, walk indoors on days when the pollen count is high.*

**Choose your route well**
*Steer clear of busy roads to reduce your exposure to car pollution.*

## Walking with osteoarthritis and osteoporosis

You might think that the more we use our joints and bones the quicker they will wear out and cause us pain. In fact, the opposite is true. Admittedly, top athletes who exercise with great intensity and put sustained pressure on their joints may well suffer wear and tear at an early age, but for most of us, the less we use our joints, the weaker the supporting muscles become, and the more our joints will wobble and wear out. Similarly, if we don't keep weight on our bones, they'll lose density and be prone to breaks.

Our joints don't like carrying a lot of extra weight. If you're both overweight and inactive, your knees or hips will start to complain, and osteoarthritis develops. It's never too late to improve your joint flexibility and strength, thus warding off and diminishing the effects of osteoarthritis, and walking is one of the best ways to do this. Regular walking also is ideal for maintaining the density of your bones, thus helping offset the effects of osteoporosis.

### A NATURAL REMEDY

The recent Fitness Arthritis and Seniors Trial (FAST), carried out by the American Medical Association, looked at the effects of aerobic exercise and resistance exercise in older adults with osteoarthritis of the knee. Participants were either encouraged to walk more, along with other physical exercise, or to carry on with their usual low level of physical activity. After one year, those who walked more felt less pain and discomfort and needed less medication and surgery than their counterparts.

If you suffer from the more serious condition of rheumatoid arthritis, you should check with your doctor before beginning a program of regular walking.

### How walking helps osteoarthritis

Osteoarthritis is the result of natural wear and tear of the joints. It usually occurs when the muscles surrounding the joint become weak due to lack of use. This allows the joint to become unstable and wear out more quickly, causing inflammation, swelling and pain. Painkillers will bring some relief, but you can do much to help your arthritis naturally, without medication.

Being overweight puts even more pressure on the joints, so a sensible diet combined with a regular

## BONE DENSITY | explained

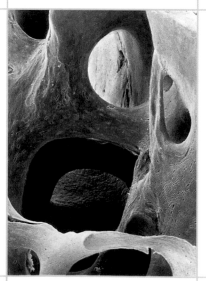

Cells, known as osteoclasts, release minerals, such as calcium, from the bones when these minerals are needed by other parts of the body. Bone mineral density (BMD) is maintained when other cells in the bones, called osteoblasts, replace these lost minerals. When BMD is normal, bones are strong and minor fractures easily repaired. In your early thirties, your body becomes less effective at replacing lost minerals and bones gradually become porous and more prone to fractures. Osteoporosis in fact means "porous bone." Bone has a honeycomb structure, as shown left. If a bone becomes osteoporotic, the honeycomb walls become thinner. Physical activity can reduce this loss of bone density, particularly load-bearing exercise, because it puts moderate pressure on the bones.

walking program will do much to relieve the pain. Thigh-muscle exercises are good because they increase the strength of the muscles that support the knee. This means the muscles rather than the joints will be taking most of the stress and strain of exercise. The knee won't wobble and the arthritis won't get worse. Acupuncture may also bring considerable relief, as may stretching and yoga. You may wish to use a cane or other support when starting out on a program of regular walking.

## How walking helps osteoporosis

This condition occurs when the density of your bones decreases. Everyone's bones start to become thinner in their early 30s, but some people suffer from osteoporosis at a much earlier age. Osteoporosis itself is painless; it's the small fractures that occur in the spine as a result of osteoporosis that cause pain and a stoop. A thinning hipbone also can increase your chances of a fracture.

Your bones are constantly developing, just like the rest of your body, and need to be exercised regularly. The critical period for bone growth is the teens and early 20s—peak bone mass is reached at the tender age of 30. Physical activity plays a crucial role in stopping the thinning of bone. If you have osteoporosis, the only physical activities that are out of bounds are contact sports and activities that present a risk of falling. The key is to increase the amount of load-bearing exercise you do. Walking is a load-bearing activity, as the bones support the "load" from the pull of the muscles and the force of gravity on the body. Bones need a variety of brief, frequent loads during the day to maintain strength and density.

You also can improve bone strength by increasing your intake of calcium and vitamin D, keeping alcohol levels down, avoiding caffeinated drinks with food, as these reduce the absorption of calcium from your food, and cutting down on salt, as this can cause the body to excrete more calcium. Women who lose a lot of weight and stop menstruating regularly don't produce enough estrogen to protect their bones, and in men who diet excessively, testosterone levels can fall very low and this causes a loss of bone density. So avoid crash diets.

*Walkers' tips*

## PROTECTING YOUR BONES

### Choose an ideal surface
*Avoid difficult terrain—stick to flat, even ground.*

### Pace yourself
*Start walking slowly and stick with this pace for as long as you want.*

### Listen to your body
*Increase the distance gradually. There's no need to rush.*

### Play safe
*Wear a bandage or other support for your inflamed joint, and take necessary painkillers at least an hour before your walk.*

### Get expert advice
*Wear good walking soles with orthotics, preferably as advised by a podiatrist.*

### Short and frequent
*Walk short distances every day rather than longer distances once a week.*

### Walk when it's warm
*Try longer walks when it's dry, sunny and warm. This weather is better for sore joints.*

### Help yourself
*Lose weight if you feel it's hampering your progress.*

### Be patient
*It will be two to three months before you start to feel the benefits.*

## Walking with diabetes

As an aerobic exercise with a low injury rate and substantial cardiovascular benefits, regular walking is one of the best treatments for diabetes. Often, diabetes can be treated simply with regular exercise and a healthy diet, sometimes preventing a progression to insulin injections. Always check with your physician before starting any new exercise program.

Diabetes is a condition that occurs when there is an upset in the careful balance of sugar (glucose) and insulin in the body. Glucose is the simple form of carbohydrates that gives us energy (see box, page 90); insulin is a hormone that helps control blood-sugar levels and is produced by special cells in the pancreas. When glucose levels rise, the pancreas produces extra insulin to remove this glucose from the bloodstream and store it in the liver. However, if the pancreas cannot produce enough insulin to maintain this balance then diabetes can occur.

- **Type 1 diabetes** This initially occurs mainly in people younger than 35. The exact cause is unknown although it's often unmasked by a viral infection which destroys insulin-producing cells, leaving the body unable to produce insulin. Children may develop high blood sugar quite suddenly and will need to start an insulin program immediately.
- **Type 2 diabetes** This occurs later in life, mainly in those 40 or older. The onset, whereby the body becomes unable to make use of or produce insulin, is more gradual than for Type 1 diabetes and may be diagnosed during a routine medical examination. Associated with obesity, it can sometimes be treated with a strict diet instead of or as well as with medication.

The combination of glucose and oxygen in our bodies releases the energy we need to work our muscles and make our bodies function properly. If the amount of glucose is too low, a hypoglycemic episode (a "hypo") can occur. This happens when blood sugar has fallen to a level at which the brain is impaired and results in weakness, confusion, dizziness and perspiring. It's usually the result of having taken too much insulin.

*Walkers' tips*

### INSULIN KNOW-HOW

#### Plan carefully
*Decide exactly when you're going to take your walk and plan your insulin injections around it. As walking uses up glucose, your normal insulin dose may be too high and you may need to compensate.*

#### Delay absorption
*If you're walking soon after an insulin injection, inject it in muscles away from the legs. This way insulin is not absorbed too quickly by the muscles that are being used during exercise, which can provoke a hypo.*

#### Check your blood sugar
*Start with a walk of about 15 minutes and monitor your blood sugar before you start and about 1 hour after you finish. If your blood sugar changes considerably, consult your doctor before tackling a longer walk.*

#### Carry glucose
*Make sure you've got liquid or tablet-form glucose with you. If there are signs of a hypo, sit down and take the glucose.*

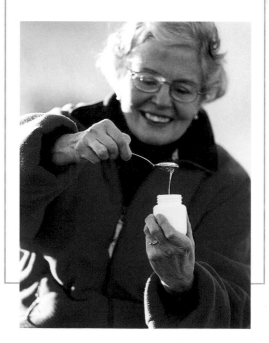

A hypo is treated quickly by taking glucose in the form of sugar-rich foods or drinks.

## How walking helps

Walking helps control your blood-sugar levels because, like any exercise, it burns up the sugar in the bloodstream through muscular activity.

If you have Type 2 diabetes, you are more prone to excess body fat, which decreases your body's sensitivity to insulin. This means that a higher dose of insulin than normal is needed to keep blood-sugar levels down. Unfortunately, increased insulin production is associated with higher blood pressure and pushes up triglycerides (a type of blood fat), which can cause heart problems. By helping you to get rid of this additional fat, walking increases your body's sensitivity to insulin, so less is needed. You also may find that insulin shots cause weight gain, so regular physical activity helps offset this too.

## The ideal amount

Try to build up to a program of at least 30 minutes a day, five days a week. The walk should be demanding enough to increase your breathing rate. This will burn up sugar, so reducing your insulin requirement and lowering cholesterol levels. Don't forget that the benefits of a walk only last a couple of days, so stick to your walking plan.

It's important to check your feet regularly when walking (see below). Feet can more easily become infected if you have diabetes, because of poor circulation and loss of sensation, so properly fitting, comfortable shoes are essential.

## Foot care

*Feet work hard while walking, so give them some attention.*

**a** Check your feet daily for cuts, blisters, sores and swelling. See your doctor about any that don't heal.

**b** Wash your feet daily in warm, not hot, water. Dry well, particularly between the toes.

**c** Smooth away corns and calluses gently using a pumice stone. Keep the skin smooth by applying skin lotion on the tops and soles of your feet, but not between the toes.

**d** Trim your toenails regularly. Cut them straight across, using clippers, not scissors, and smooth the edges with an emery board.

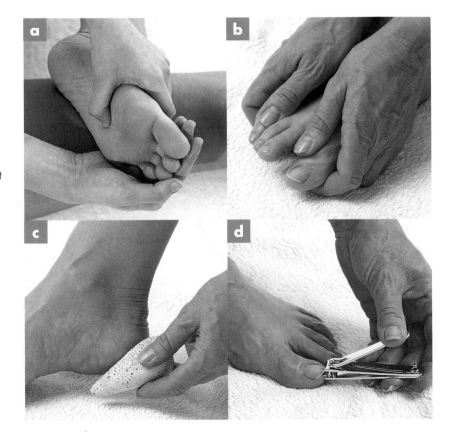

# FIRST AID

*It makes sense for a committed walker to be equipped
with a basic first-aid kit and know how to use its
contents. This section describes the most common
complaints and tells you how to give basic treatment.*

Walking is one of the safest forms of exercise. Our bodies were designed to walk, so we should find it a completely natural and injury-free activity. However, as with any physical exercise, there are some risks involved. It is always advisable to have a first-aid kit at home, and to take one out on walks of more than a couple of hours or so, particularly if you are with a group. These pages also tell you how to deal with many of the more common minor injuries and a few of the more serious ones you might encounter while walking.

## Preventing falls

Uneven and challenging terrain is the cause of many falls while walking, but they can be a result of poor fitness also. Fortunately, most falls can be prevented simply by watching where you walk and avoiding or slowing down over tricky spots. This is why it helps to familiarize yourself with your route before walking it at a fast pace. Skirt around slippery patches of ice and snow and wet grass, leaves or moss if you feel nervous. If you're in a park or wood, keep an eye out for rocks, tree roots and holes dug by animals. In cities, uneven or crumbling sidewalks are more of a problem, and you should be careful around areas that are being dug up or repaired. Dogs, particularly large friendly ones, may be a hazard if they jump and surprise you.

Sometimes falls are caused by internal factors—a result of poor balance or flexibility or weak joints or muscles. Walking should help you improve your fitness in all of these areas, and you can help yourself further by stretching regularly (see pages 39 to 41) and performing specific exercises (see pages 178 to 181). Similarly, if you do fall, you'll recover more quickly.

## The first-aid kit

The basic supplies for walking are outlined in the box, opposite, and these are all that's needed for most situations. Even if most of your walks last less than an

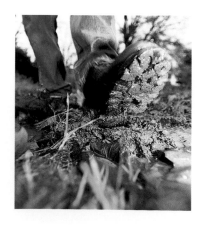

## PREVENTING FALLS ▶▶▶ ▶▶ ▶▶ ▶▶

Although it is sometimes necessary to slow down on slippery or uneven terrain, taking very small steps and placing each foot gingerly is likely to compromise your balance, causing you to slip and fall. Instead, stride out with confidence. Each time you place your heel down, do so forcefully and positively. Most twigs and soft mud will yield to your body weight and you can keep walking with your natural rhythm and balance. If you wear shoes or boots with a deep tread and patterns in various directions on the soles, this will also help prevent slipping.

hour and you don't feel that you need to take one along with you, you should at least have such a kit at home. If you buy a ready-packaged kit from a shop, check that it contains all the items. Extra supplies, such as blister materials, insect repellent and bite creams, can be useful if you expect to encounter any of the hazards discussed in the rest of this chapter.

For walks lasting a day or longer, or when you are venturing into extreme weather or environments, you will need a more comprehensive kit, specifically geared to your needs. You may, for example, consider taking flares, splints, a blanket and a flashlight. Ask at your outdoor-equipment store for advice.

Many bandages and first-aid items include instructions for use. You should familiarize yourself, however, with the contents of a first-aid manual and keep it at home in an easily accessible place in case of emergency, or, even better, go on a first-aid course.

### Safety first

Take extra care with anti-inflammatories, such as ibuprofen, or painkillers, such as acetaminophen. Anti-inflammatories can be dangerous if taken by some asthma sufferers, as they can cause an attack. Painkillers should not be given to someone who has collapsed or may need surgery—for example, for a broken bone—as surgery can only be carried out on an individual who has had nothing to eat or drink for the previous 4 hours.

## Foot and nail problems

Your feet are the parts of your body most vulnerable to injury when walking. Below we cover some of the most frequently occurring conditions associated with walking and advice on how they can be prevented and treated.

### Blisters

One of the most common complaints associated with walking, blisters only really become a problem once you've started to walk longer distances. They are caused by friction that occurs when your sweaty skin is rubbed by your footwear.

---

### ✔ WHAT DO I NEED IN A KIT?

- ❑ **Adhesive dressings** Include a variety of shapes and sizes in your kit for use on minor wounds.
- ❑ **Non-adhesive dressings** Make sure that these are sterile and that you have a few different sizes.
- ❑ **Sling** This is not only for breaks and sprains, but also for elevating cut arms or hands.
- ❑ **Elastic bandage** Use this or a tubular grip for supporting sprains and holding dressings in place.
- ❑ **Safety pins** Use these or clips to secure bandages.
- ❑ **Adhesive tape** Use this to fix dressings in place. Some people may be allergic to some types.
- ❑ **Gauze pads** Include a pack of 10, for use as dressings, padding or swabs.
- ❑ **Antiseptic towelettes** Use these on small wounds.
- ❑ **Antibiotic cream** This prevents infections.
- ❑ **Antihistamines** These can reduce a reaction to bites and stings.
- ❑ **Scissors** Make sure that these are blunt-ended.
- ❑ **Space blanket** This is a silver-foil blanket that retains heat.
- ❑ **Whistle** This is a great way to draw attention.

---

One of the best ways of avoiding blisters is by making sure your shoes fit well. When you walk long distances your feet will expand, so your walking shoes should be half a size larger than your normal shoes (see page 123). Check that there are no seams rubbing the areas where blisters might form. When you use new shoes make sure you break them in slowly so that they can form to the shape of your foot and become less stiff.

If the skin on your feet is tough and painless, resist using pumice stones or skin softeners, as this hard skin will prevent you from getting blisters in these areas. If

## THE RICE PRINCIPLE

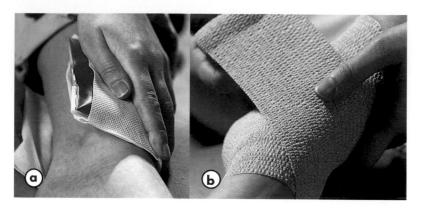

To treat sprains, rest the injured area, cover it with ice **a**, such as frozen peas or packed snow, then fit a compression bandage to reduce swelling **b**. Finally elevate the area. Remember:

**Rest**

**Ice**

**Compression**

**Elevation**

the skin is dry, cracked and painful, however, then rub a skin softening cream into the area after you wash to relieve any soreness.

As you walk, keep your feet dry by wearing socks that wick moisture away from the skin (see page 127). Thin liner socks beneath your normal socks are ideal, as the friction occurs between the socks rather than between the sock and your skin. On a long walk, carry spare socks to change into if your feet get damp.

If you do get a blister, cover the area with adhesive bandage or blister material. There are several types of blister materials, with various brand names. Moleskin, and other adhesive dressings, consist of plastic or soft fabric with an adhesive back, which protects against further friction on the affected area. Spenco 2nd Skin, and other blister pads, are soft, liquid-gel pads, which cushion the area. These may be held in place using first-aid tape or duct tape. Carry blister materials with you on a long walk or when breaking in a pair of new shoes. Always treat a "hot spot" as soon as you notice it, to stop a blister from forming.

If you have a small blister, the best policy is to do nothing—it will soon fade away. In fact, it will harden the skin as it heals. If it's a large blister, it might be best to drain it. First, wipe the skin with alcohol, and then wipe a needle as well to sterilize it. Drain it using gentle pressure and cover the area with a bandage. Do not peel skin away, as it will protect the raw underlayer.

### Plantar fasciitis (heel pain)

A result of weight gain or of wearing shoes that have little "spring" left in them, this is a condition that can become very painful during a walk. The plantar fascia is a long band of fibers extending from the bottom of the heel bone to the base of the toes. Due to its position, it takes quite a battering when we walk. If the fibers become irritated or inflamed, pain occurs deep in the heel pad, and it can feel like a rock in your shoe. The pain is worse in the morning, because the plantar fascia shortens and tightens during the night. People with flat feet, high arches and tight Achilles tendons are particularly prone to this condition.

The pain can last for up to six months but usually goes away on its own before then. To prevent and ease this condition, wear well-fitting shoes and use orthotics or heel inserts that absorb shock. Try to keep your walks shorter and on soft ground. Practicing the RICE principle (see box, above) will bring some relief, as will stretching the calf muscles and the muscles and tendons of the foot. To stretch your foot, wrap a towel around your toes, hold the two ends and pull your toes toward you.

### Metatarsalgia (forefoot pain)

This is a general term to denote pain in the ball of the foot (the metatarsal region) that can sometimes feel like lots of small stones in your shoes. It's a common condition and occurs when the joints and tendons just below the base of the toes become inflamed, usually because of a long period of excessive pressure—it is a particular problem of women who spend long periods in high-heeled shoes. As with plantar fasciitis, the best way to cure it is to stop wearing the shoes that may be causing the problem. Wear low-heeled shoes that bend at the ball of the foot and have a wide toe box to allow your toes to spread out. Orthotic insoles and pads can spread the weight more evenly over your feet and bring significant relief from pain.

### Ingrown toenail

This is a painful condition caused by wearing ill-fitting shoes that squeeze the toes or by cutting your toenail incorrectly. It usually occurs on the big toe, and the pain is a result of the nail cutting into the skin at either side of it. There may be associated redness, bleeding and infection. Walking can aggravate the pain.

Treat sore and inflamed toes by bathing them in warm salt water then covering the nail in a gauze dressing. When cutting your toenails, make sure you cut in a straight line as opposed to curving the edges.

### Black toenail

This occurs when a blood blister forms beneath your toenail, because you have stubbed it, dropped something on it or because your toe butts up against the end of your shoe. Walkers are particularly prone to black toenails when walking downhill. If your nail does turn black, it may fall off. However, it will probably grow back again without any permanent damage. If it is very painful, see a doctor, who can safely drain the blood from under your nail.

To prevent black toenails, consider the following:
- **Good shoes** Make sure that your feet are pulled back from the front of the toe box when you tighten the laces (see page 123). Some specialist shops have slopes on which you can test the fit.
- **Thick socks** Wear good, thick socks or two pairs of socks to prevent your toes from hitting the ends of your shoes. Also choose socks that keep your feet dry so that they don't slide around too much.

*Walkers' tips*

## BLITZ THOSE BLISTERS

### Keep them dry
*Wear socks that wick moisture away from the foot, and change socks when they get damp. Also, dust your feet with talcum powder or apply underarm antiperspirant.*

### Lubricate the area
*Reduce friction by rubbing feet with petroleum jelly or barrier cream. Reapply this every hour on long walks.*

### Cover it up
*Protect a blister or "hot spot" with blister materials or adhesive bandages.*

### Double up
*Wear two pairs of socks: thin liner socks under your regular socks.*

### Do nothing
*If you do get a blister the best thing to do is leave it alone and let it heal itself.*

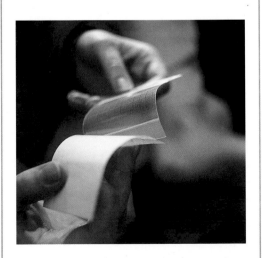

■ **Lace locks** Fasten your laces as for a narrow foot (see page 125), as this prevents the bottom half of your laces loosening.

■ **Orthotics** Insoles that support the arches of your feet will help prevent your feet sliding forward.

■ **Taping your toes** Wrap your toes in duct tape or first-aid tape to relieve pressure on them.

## Athlete's foot

This is a fungus that appears as patches of red, flaky, itchy skin, particularly between the third and fourth, and/or fourth and fifth toes. The skin can sometimes crack painfully. Walkers often suffer from athlete's foot because the fungus thrives in the warm, moist atmosphere of the inside of your shoe. Your pharmacist should be able to offer you special talcum powders, creams and sprays to treat the condition.

Minimize your chances of developing athlete's foot. Keep your feet clean and dry thoroughly, especially between the toes. Change your socks and shoes often. If appropriate, wear walking sandals to allow air between your toes.

## Corns and calluses

These are very similar conditions, consisting of an accumulation of hard, dead skin cells on the foot. They are a result of regular friction or pressure on an area and are often caused by ill-fitting shoes. Corns usually appear on the toes, while calluses are more common on the heels or the balls of your feet. Many corns, and some calluses, have a core that can press on the nerves causing pain. For most people, neither condition is serious, and they can be relieved by changing your shoes and using pads or orthotics that relieve pressure on the affected area. Resist the temptation to cut away the hard skin, as it can make the problem worse. If you are diabetic, see your doctor with any foot condition.

## Muscles, joints and bones

You run the risk of straining your muscles or injuring your tendons or joints if you push yourself too quickly or are not warming up before a fast walk. There are several conditions to which walkers are prone.

## Muscle strains

These usually occur in the calves or the muscles at the back of the thigh (the hamstrings). The muscle itself will feel tender when you apply pressure. Most strains are not serious and you can continue to walk slowly. Keep the muscle warm by using muscle rubs or a hot-water bottle or heating pad. Take an anti-inflammatory if necessary. The condition usually rights itself within two weeks, but if it continues or prevents you from walking then you may have a partial muscle tear and should see a doctor.

## Stiffness

If you really push yourself on a long or fast walk, you may feel it the next morning. Taking arnica tablets or an anti-inflammatory may help but, better still, end the problem before it even starts by warming up and cooling down correctly (see pages 34 to 41). Also, take it easy for a day or two after a strenuous walk to give the small tears time to heal.

## Twisted or sprained ankle

This is a risk if you're walking on uneven ground, particularly if you have weak ankles or have suffered a sprained ankle in the past. Minimize your risk by protecting the area with a support bandage, available at drugstores or sporting-goods stores, or by wearing boots that come high up the ankle and have a strong toe box (see page 124).

There are three levels of ankle injury. A first-degree injury is when ligaments stretch but do not tear. There will be some pain on movement but little swelling or bruising. You can carry on walking and the pain should go within about a week. Second-degree ankle injuries are when the ligaments are partially torn. There is swelling and bruising and you'll probably be limping. Healing can take up to six weeks. Third-degree injuries are complete ligament tears. You won't be able to move your foot and swelling will be intense. You'll probably hear a snap when the injury occurs and you may require surgery. Whatever your level of injury, practicing the RICE principle (see page 110) as soon as possible will minimize swelling and pain.

## TREATING CRAMPS

These painful muscle spasms can occur after exercise due to a buildup of chemicals in the muscles or loss of salt and water through sweating. Stretching out the muscle and exercise will help ease the pain. For foot cramps, stretch out the sole of the foot by standing with your weight on your toes. For calf cramps, sit down, straighten your leg and slowly pull your toes toward you to stretch the calf. It can help to have a friend push gently on your toes. For cramps in the backs of your thighs, lie down and raise your leg. Straighten your leg gently and massage the muscle.

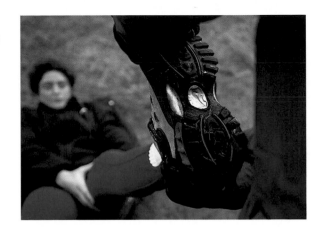

### Shinsplints

This is a general term that refers to pain of the lower leg, which occurs just below the knee (see also page 55). The pain usually comes on gradually and recedes when you rest. The condition is generally a result of stepping up the pace too quickly or introducing hills to your walks before you're ready. To prevent the problem, reduce your walking, make sure that you wear good shoes, warm up and cool down properly (see pages 34 to 41) and check your technique (see pages 25 to 27).

### Tendinitis

This condition is a little more serious than a muscle strain. It manifests itself as a feeling of tenderness over an area of bone, such as the side of the knee, hip or Achilles tendon. It generally comes on slowly and may be accompanied by redness and swelling.

Tendinitis is generally caused by overuse or may also be caused by a lack of symmetry in your posture—for example, if one leg is slightly shorter than the other—and this creates tension at the point at which the tendon joins the bone. It can also occur if you begin an exercise program when you are unused to exercise. If you are experiencing pain after two weeks, consult your doctor, who will treat the immediate problem. Long-term treatment may involve specially designed orthotics to correct your posture.

### Stress fractures

These are small cracks in the outer layer of a bone in the foot and occur if you've been pushing yourself too hard, too fast, particularly if you're walking on hard surfaces. If you feel a specific spot of sharp pain when you run your hand along your shin, or experience swelling and pain in the front part of your foot, you probably have a stress fracture. A horizontal rather than a vertical line of pain is another indicator. You'll need a bone scan for a proper diagnosis. The fracture will probably heal on its own with adequate rest, but you may need a cast. To prevent stress fractures make sure you increase your training gradually and replace your shoes before they're too worn (see page 126).

## Skin problems

Your skin can become easily irritated by such factors as your clothes, the sun or poisonous plants while out walking, particularly in hot weather. These conditions are rarely serious and can usually be treated at home.

### Chafing

This occurs when clothing or skin rubs sweating skin. Sweat, if concentrated, can be a considerable irritant, so make sure you drink adequately on any walk. Use talcum powder to reduce friction and keep the skin dry. If you apply a deodorant, make it a dry stick rather than a liquid roll-on, which can make the skin sticky. Another good tip is to apply petroleum jelly (Vaseline), particularly under the arms and between the thighs.

## Sunburn

There's no excuse to suffer from sunburn, because it is easily avoided. Cover up with clothes and apply sunscreen of at least SPF 15 for adults and SPF 30 for children before going out. Don't forget the ears, nose, back of the neck, backs of the legs and top of the head (or wear a hat). These spots are often overlooked and can be painful if they burn. Remember that you can burn on cloudy days. Treat sunburn immediately with calamine lotion, cool compresses or aloe vera gel. Drink plenty of fluids and stay cool.

## Plant rashes

Though rarely serious, a rash from stinging nettles, pollen or fungal spores can be irritating. If you do get stung, antihistamine cream should relieve the itching and redness, and symptoms should subside within a few hours. Dock leaves can bring immediate relief from stinging nettles, because the sting contains an acid, and the dock leaf contains an alkali.

Poison ivy, poison oak and poison sumac have poisonous sap that can cause itching, redness and burning of the skin a day or two after contact. You can be affected if you touch clothes or pets that have come into contact with the sap. You may be able to prevent a reaction by doing the following within 6 hours:

- Remove all clothes and equipment that have come into contact with the sap.
- Wash your skin with soap and cold water.
- Using cotton balls, rub alcohol onto the affected parts of your skin.

If a reaction does occur, then you may be able to treat yourself with calamine lotion, baking soda and water paste or antihistamine cream. Try not to scratch the skin. If self-treatment fails, see your doctor.

## Cuts and bruises

If you suffer a small cut, clean it with soap and water and apply antiseptic cream before covering it with an adhesive bandage. If the bleeding is fairly heavy, use firm pressure and hold a bandage over the cut for 10 minutes as you elevate the area to slow blood flow. If the bleeding continues, wrap the cut tightly, without restricting the blood supply and seek medical advice.

Most bruises are harmless and no treatment is needed. Arnica cream or tablets may be useful in reducing the pain and severity of bruising. You can reduce some of the discoloration with vitamin K cream. If you have a very large bruise that is hard, painful and is darker than normal, then blood may be trapped in the muscle and medical advice should be sought.

## REMOVING BITE VENOM

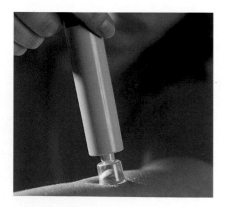

Special pumps are available that can quickly draw out venom left by a bite or sting. These function by way of a vacuum that quickly sucks into your skin. They are effective against wasp and bee stings, mosquito, ant, spider and snake bites, and are safe to use on children. The pumps usually come with a number of extractor cups in different sizes, so you can select the best cup size for the type of wound. It's important to note that these devices will remove only the poison (i.e. the liquid), not the stinger itself, which will need to be drawn out with tweezers. Use the pump immediately after a bite or sting, but always seek medical advice as well if you feel that the reaction is severe.

## Bites and stings

The bites and stings from insects, marine creatures and snakes introduce a chemical or venom that can be painful and cause the skin to swell and itch. These bites also carry the risk of allergic reactions and infections. For all bites, your priority is to wash the area with soap and water before applying antibiotic cream and a bandage. On stings, use ice to calm the swelling and an antihistamine cream to ease irritation. You can also use a venom remover (see box, opposite) on certain types of sting. These measures will help reduce pain and swelling, but medical attention must be sought if there is an infection or allergic reaction—indicated by swelling or difficulty breathing (see box, right).

Minimize your risk by wearing long-sleeved tops and pants, instead of shorts, and by applying insect repellent containing the chemical DEET to skin and clothes. Essential oils such as citronella, cedar oil, eucalyptus and rosemary can help. Avoid perfumes, colognes or hair spray, as these can attract insects.

### Bee stings

If you or a fellow walker are stung you must first remove the stinger, if it's still in the skin. Pull it out gently with tweezers or a fingernail. Try not to squeeze it, as this will release more venom into the skin. Wash the affected area and apply antibiotic cream. Minimize pain and swelling with an ice bag. If you're not allergic, irritation will be minimal. To avoid tempting bees, don't wear strong-smelling toiletries or bright clothing.

### Spider bites

Bites from certain spiders, such as black widow, can cause nausea, fever and, in extreme cases, be fatal. If you receive a spider bite you should keep the bitten area still and hanging down. Wash as normal and apply an ice bag before seeking medical attention. You may be prescribed antibiotics.

### Ticks

These are a risk because ticks can carry Lyme disease. This may be a serious condition so medical attention should be sought as soon as possible if you receive a

**SAFETY FIRST**

Though most stings are relatively harmless, there is a risk that they can cause anaphylactic shock—a major allergic reaction that is potentially fatal. Symptoms occur within minutes and include: swelling of the face and neck, difficulty breathing and red, blotchy skin. Phone for medical assistance immediately. Some people are aware of their susceptibility and carry a syringe of adrenaline (Epi-Pen), which you can help inject.

tick bite. Never use your finger to remove a tick as this can spread infection. Brush it away using a stone or stick. If you are in an area known for Lyme disease you can usually protect yourself by getting vaccinated.

### Snake bites

Of the hundreds of different kinds of snakes naturally found in North America, only four types are poisonous: coral snakes, copperheads, rattlesnakes, and water moccasins or cottonmouths. Copperheads, rattlesnakes, and water moccasins are all pit vipers—thick, heavy snakes that inject venom, usually with a single bite. Coral snakes are comparatively small and thin and usually bite the fingers or toes.

If a fellow walker is bitten by a poisonous snake, call for medical help immediately. If this is not nearby, begin treatment until help arrives. Never cut open the skin around a bite or use suction to try to remove venom unless directed to do so by an emergency dispatcher, and never suck venom from a wound with your mouth. Snake venom causes tissue damage, breathing difficulties, dizziness, nausea, headache and, perhaps most importantly, shock. Look for signs of shock including cold, clammy skin; blue-tinged or pale skin; dazed expression, weak rapid pulse; shallow breathing; and weakness. Lay the victim down, keeping the bitten limb immobile and lower than the level of the heart. Remove any constricting items and maintain the body temperature until help arrives.

## Major medical problems

We all have the responsibility to learn everything we can about the more serious conditions that could affect us or our fellow walkers. The likelihood of any of these conditions occurring on your walk is extremely low, but knowing what to do in case of an emergency could save a life. Consider signing up for first-aid training.

### Heat exhaustion

When we exercise we produce sweat, which evaporates and cools our skin. If we overexert ourselves on hot and humid days, however, the loss of water and salt through excessive sweating can lead to heat exhaustion. Symptoms are headaches, sickness, cool, clammy skin, a dry mouth, muscle cramps, dizziness, and eventual collapse. The treatment is straightforward: Get out of the sun, replenish fluids and salts, and try to cool off.

### Heatstroke

This is a more serious condition that is often the result of untreated heat exhaustion. It can strike suddenly. Sweating stops and the body can no longer be cooled by evaporation. Body temperature rises rapidly to levels of 113°F (45°C). When a person experiences heatstroke he or she becomes very confused and dizzy, has a rapid pulse, dilated pupils and hot and dry skin. The victim may also experience hallucinations and convulsions and collapse into unconsciousness.

You need to cool the person down as rapidly as possible. Remove clothing and cover the person with a cold, wet sheet. If you do not have a sheet, then fan the victim and sponge him or her with cold water. Be prepared to use CPR if necessary (see box, below). Once the victim's temperature drops to a safe level—below 100.4°F (38°C)—continue to monitor him or her carefully until help arrives.

### Hypothermia

This occurs as a result of a dramatic fall in body temperature, but is unlikely to happen unless you're injured or unable to move or because you become wet through in cold and windy conditions. In a person suffering from hypothermia, blood will be rerouted from the extremities to the trunk to keep vital organs warm and full of blood. The victim will initially shiver, as the body temperature falls below 95°F (35°C), and then become drowsy and confused. You should treat a victim in the following way:

## CPR | explained

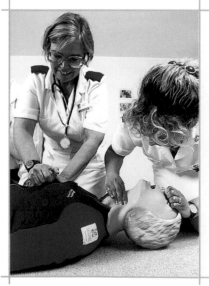

Cardiopulmonary resuscitation (CPR), consisting of mouth-to-mouth breathing and chest compressions, is one of the most important lifesaving techniques you can learn. It can be vital to save life if a major medical emergency occurs on a long hike, where you may be walking in an isolated area far from medical help and amenities. If you're a walking group leader, then CPR training is compulsory. Proper first-aid training can only be taught by a fully qualified instructor. Contact the American Red Cross or the Canadian Red Cross for a list of certified CPR courses, or check out the bulletin board in your community health center. All-purpose courses usually include techniques for treating other serious conditions such as fractures, hypothermia and shock.

- **Remove wet clothing** Then immediately wrap the person in dry clothing.
- **Give him or her warm drinks** This will bring the internal body temperature up.
- **Move gently** If you try to get to shelter, move the victim slowly and carefully.
- **Warm the victim in any way** Keep the person as dry, sheltered and warm as possible, even using your own body heat if you are not putting yourself at risk. Do not give the victim your clothes, as you will put yourself at risk.

## Bone fractures

The most likely broken bones experienced when walking are those of the wrist, hip, leg or ankle. Even a fracture as mild as one in the wrist can still cause shock (see below) so keep the person warm and still while you call for help. A more serious fracture is that of the hip or leg. The person usually experiences a lot of pain if moved, but the pain might disappear when he or she is lying still. An obvious sign of hip fracture is that when the victim is lying down one leg appears shorter than the other and the foot is turned out. Call for help and keep the person warm with a space blanket. Do not give the person anything to eat or drink.

## Shock

A person is in medical shock when his or her blood pressure falls dramatically. This can be caused by internal bleeding, an infection in the bloodstream, a wound, a broken bone or dehydration. The person will have cold, clammy, blue-gray skin and a fast but weak pulse, followed by weakness, giddiness and nausea. Eventually the victim may gasp for air, collapse and become unconscious.

To treat shock, lay the person down on a blanket with his or her legs propped up to keep the blood supply flowing to the brain. Undo any tight clothing that restricts the neck, chest or waist and keep the person warm with layers of clothes and a space blanket. Call for medical assistance immediately.

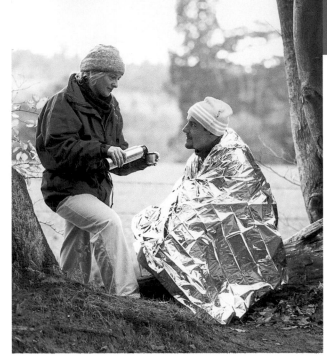

**Hypothermia**
*Wrap the person in a silver-foil space blanket to retain heat and talk calmly and reassuringly until help arrives.*

---

### ✔ WHAT DETAILS DO I NEED?

- ❑ **Where** Tell the operator exactly where to find the person needing help, including road and junction names, landmarks or map details.

- ❑ **Who** Give the operator the name of the casualty, as well as the person's sex and age, and give your name.

- ❑ **How** Provide brief details of what has caused the condition or injury.

- ❑ **What** Give as many details as you can about the condition of the casualty, including what you think he or she is suffering from and whether the casualty is conscious and/or breathing.

- ❑ **When** Let the operator know how long it has taken you to get in contact.

- ❑ **Contact details** Leave your telephone number and location in case the operator needs to contact you.

# **HEALTH** TROUBLESHOOTER

*Walking is safe for almost anyone, but do check with your doctor before you start a program. This section looks at some typical health questions people have.*

**I have rheumatoid arthritis. Can I safely take up walking?**

Rheumatoid arthritis is a very different condition from osteoarthritis, and it's not advised to walk when your joints are particularly inflamed. Rest your joints when you have a flare-up—increased activity will only make them more painful.

**I have a heart condition and would like to know if it's dangerous to start walking.**

Walking is the safest form of physical activity. However, if you have any of the following symptoms, it would be advised to see your doctor before you start walking:

▶ Chest (or upper body) discomfort that is brought on by exertion
▶ Difficulty breathing during exertion
▶ Dizziness or nausea during exertion
▶ Faint feeling during or just after physical activity
▶ Palpitations (fast or irregular heartbeat) during activity

**I have not exercised for many years but now want to start. What will my doctor ask me when assessing whether I am fit enough?**

Your doctor should be aware of your medical history. If not, he or she will ask you whether you've had a major illness such as a recent blood clot, diabetes or heart problem, and whether there is any family history of cardiomyopathy (a rare inherited disease of the heart muscle). Your doctor will then take your pulse and blood pressure, listen to your heart for a murmur, listen to your lungs for fluid and order a blood test and perhaps an electrocardiogram (ECG) just to be sure.

**I have heard that it's not advisable for athletes to train when their throats are sore. Does this apply to walkers?**

It's true that athletes who overtrain when they have sore throats can suffer weakened immune systems and continuous viral infections. Walking is less strenuous than running, so it's fine to walk with a sore throat. The general rule is that if you have an illness that affects the neck and up (tickle in the throat, headache), walking poses no problems, but if your illness is rooted farther down (such as a chest cough), you should check with your physician.

**Which conditions should I discuss with my doctor before taking up walking?**

There are a few conditions that are incompatible with walking. Use this list as a guide, but if you're at all unsure, consult your doctor to discuss it further.

► Unstable angina (angina that is getting worse)
► Aortic stenosis (a narrowing of the aortic valve)
► A recent stroke, heart attack or a blood clot in the lung or in the leg
► Poorly controlled epilepsy
► A recent operation (last 3 months)
► Any irregular heartbeat, particularly if this is brought on by activity
► Myocarditis or pericarditis (infection of the heart muscle from a virus)
► Unstable diabetes (when the blood-sugar level is difficult to control)
► Inflamed joints from rheumatoid and other forms of inflammatory arthritis (not osteoarthritis)
► Very high blood pressure (more than 190/100)
► Any illness still undiagnosed

**I am taking some drugs to control my blood pressure and cholesterol. Do I need advice before starting to walk?**

Physical activity rarely affects the efficiency of drugs, and likewise drugs generally don't hinder your ability to perform physical activity. If taking beta-blockers, your heartbeat will be slower than normal when active. This does not mean you can't continue walking, but it won't be an accurate measure of your fitness. If taking a blood thinner, then pay particular attention to any cuts or bruises—the blood loss may actually be greater than it seems, because of the thinness of the blood.

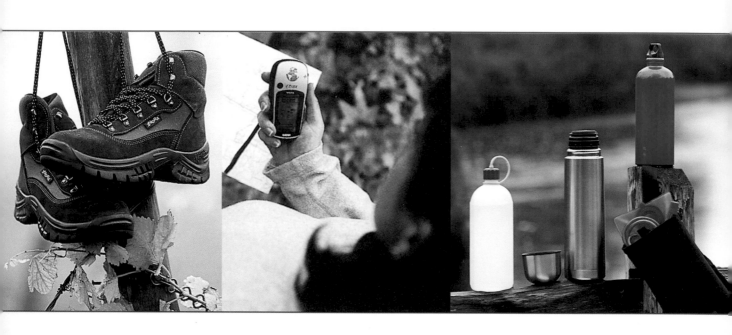

# EQUIPMENT

*The shoes, clothing and accessories you need to ensure you are walking safely and comfortably and to help you improve your technique.*

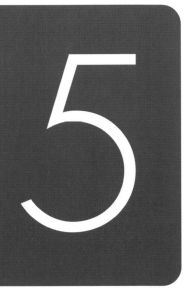

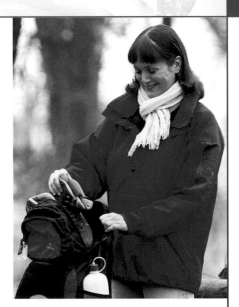

# GETTING IN **GEAR**

*Now that you've decided to take to the trails, it's time to consider the equipment that will make your walking experience comfortable and enjoyable. This chapter guides you through clothing, footwear and accessories.*

When choosing clothing and equipment, you need to consider the weather conditions, terrain, and type of walking they will be used for. In the summer months, you should be in light, synthetic materials that wick away moisture from the skin (see page 76). In winter, you should dress in layers with a waterproof jacket and a fleece vest or pullover underneath (see page 78). A series of layers will keep you warm and prevent overheating. Shoes and boots should give sufficient support, but let the feet breathe.

If you're a gadget addict, there are plenty of nifty accessories available, such as water bottles and flasks, fanny packs, pedometers, heart-rate monitors and trekking poles. These respond to your different needs during a walk: Some are there to maximize efficiency and comfort; others provide a quick "progress check;" and others, such as walking sticks and poles, give you a helping hand on your walk.

## Where to shop
Local outdoor-equipment stores are a good place to start looking for walking gear. Whether part of a major chain or privately owned, specialty stores have a range of clothing, footwear and accessories, as well as knowledgeable and helpful staff. Some manufacturers have outlet stores, where you'll be able to buy decent equipment for less. Larger department stores are another option, though the salespeople may not have any expertise about the products.

### Get on the Net
The Internet is a great place to shop in comfort. Most major outdoor-equipment companies have their own websites. If you don't have any particular manufacturer in mind, then simply type in "outdoor equipment" in a search engine and this will take you to a range of useful sites. From there you should find addresses and

## Basic equipment
You don't need lots of gear to take up walking. The basics are: a pullover or fleece that's light enough to carry, but will keep you warm; shoes that are comfortable and suited to the terrain; a day pack so that you can keep your arms and hands free; and a foldable waterproof jacket that fits in your bag.

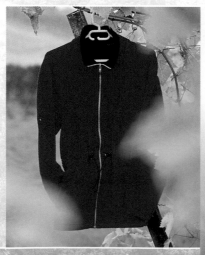

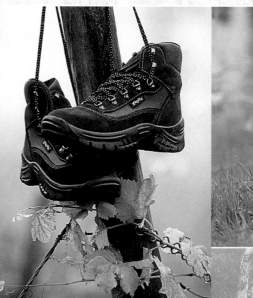

contact numbers of outlets in your area. Many companies sell their equipment over the Net, which can save you time and frustration if there are no stores nearby. But some items are better to buy in person, after trying on for fit, particularly when it comes to footwear. If you'd rather not shop online, the Internet can still be useful for finding product information before visiting a store.

## Mail order

This is another good way to "browse before you buy" and is particularly good if you're looking for out-of-season clothing, because mail-order companies carry year-round stock. REI, L.L. Bean and Campmor are among the most popular and frequently updated catalogs, with prices that tend to be competitive. Again, you'll need to be sure of your size when you order.

## Which is my brand?

It's never a bad idea to look at major brands—they are usually successful for a reason. However, this doesn't mean you should rule out other manufacturers just because their names are unfamiliar. Some of the smaller manufacturers make great gear, and their informed staff can be particularly helpful in pointing you in the right direction.

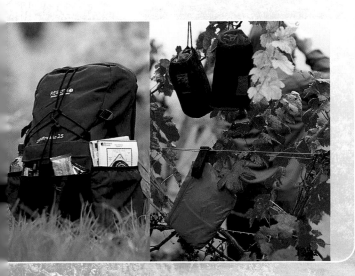

## Footwear

Comfort is the most important factor when choosing footwear. Of course, style and color are what make a particular boot or shoe appealing, but neglect comfort and your stylish shoe will quickly lose its attraction.

It's best not to use your sneakers or running shoes for walking, unless you're just going to the store and back. For a rundown of what to look for in walking shoes and boots, see page 126.

## Size matters

The correct size of your walking shoes or boots may not be the same as your normal dress-shoe size. This is because walking for an hour or so can cause your feet to swell by up to half a size. Therefore, it's best to try on boots or shoes late in the day, when your feet will have been "working" for a while.

When trying on footwear, test the fit of one shoe at a time. With the shoes unlaced, stand up and tap the toe of one shoe on the ground to slide your foot to the front. While your foot rests on the toe, there should be space to slip your finger between your heel and the back of the shoe. Tighten the laces and your foot will be pulled back a bit. Now your heel should not move more than ½ in. (1 cm) in any direction. However, the shoe should not be too tight at the heel, as it could give you blisters. You should have room in the toe box to wiggle your toes—this prevents your toes from butting against the front of the shoe when walking downhill. Also, you should be able to comfortably flex your foot and ankle. Women's shoes tend to have heels that are softer or V-shaped, because women's Achilles tendons are exposed lower on the ankle than men's.

Ill-fitting shoes can lead to problems such as blisters or black toenails (see page 110). If your shoes are too loose and your heels are lifting, add flat insoles. The insoles (or sockliners) should be replaced a couple of times during the life of your shoes, because they lose their shape and ability to cushion and support the foot.

## Fabrics for feet

When choosing your shoes, consider the materials. Generally speaking, natural products, such as leather, are kinder to feet than synthetic ones, and this is largely because they allow the foot to "breathe." Rubber soles have "spring" to protect the feet from jarring and provide good grip on slippery ground. Some synthetic materials, however, do have advantages. Uppers made of nylon and Cordura, for example, are flexible. In combination with full-grain leather they fit the foot shape well. Synthetic materials also are lightweight, inexpensive and breathable, so they release excess heat. A Gore-Tex layer makes synthetic and leather footwear waterproof, but it also raises the price.

## Lacing techniques

Buying the correct shoe size is your first priority, but you can actually solve some fitting problems by adjusting the lacing. Always loosen the laces as you slip on your shoes to prevent stress on the eyelets, and never have your laces too long, because they could

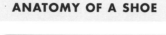

**ANATOMY OF A SHOE**

**Upper** This portion of the shoe, around the sides and top of the foot, should be flexible but also rigid enough to offer support.

**Tongue** Protecting the foot from the laces, this should be well padded. To prevent rain getting in, choose a bellows tongue—one with a flap attaching the tongue to the upper.

**Eyelets** The more eyelets, the easier you'll be able to adjust the fit. Some boots have "locking" eyelets on the ankles allowing you to adjust the foot and ankle separately.

**Stitching** With fewer seams, a shoe will last longer and be resistant to leakage.

**Rand** This protects the join of the upper and the outsole, improving durability and waterproofing.

**Insole (sockliner)** For cushioning and comfort. Good insoles stabilize the heel and support the arch.

**Midsole** A soft midsole offers comfort on flat, even ground, while a stiff midsole protects on rocky paths.

**Outsole** The bottom of the shoe needs to be solid enough to protect your foot from stones. If you can press your thumb into it, it may be too soft.

**Tread** Deeper treads will give you more traction.

**Toe box** This varies in width to suit your foot. For rocky paths, choose a toe box with a high, solid rand.

## LACING TO FIT

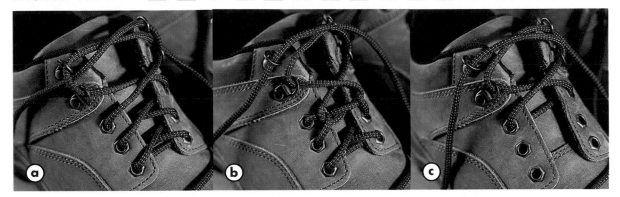

**To prevent heel slipping** Lace as normal up to the second-to-the-last eyelet. Then lace directly to the last eyelet on the same side to form two loops. Take each lace to the opposite side and slip them through the loops you've created **a.**

**For narrow feet** Do the "lace lock" as with the technique to prevent heel slipping, but create the loops in the middle eyelets. Lace as normal to the top **b.** If your shoes have two or more sets of eyelets, use the outer eyelets for a snug fit.

**For wide feet** If your forefoot is wide, leave the first few eyelets unlaced **c.** If your foot is wide over your arch miss out one or two sets of eyelets in the middle of the shoe.

cause you to trip. The conventional method of lacing, crisscross to the top of the shoe, works best for the majority of people, though adaptations can help with certain fit problems (see box, above).

### Insoles and orthotics

Walking shoes all come with their own removable insoles (also called sockliners). These offer some shock absorption, but you may find that you need a greater level of support, particularly if you have a low arch or the balls or heels of your feet often feel sore. If so, replace your sockliners with one of the following:

■ **Foam-cushioning soles** These are particularly good for older walkers, because the soles of your feet often thin with age.

■ **Orthotic insoles** These are ready-made insoles that mold to your foot, supporting your arches and providing cushioning.

Both types of insole can be bought over the counter. Custom-made orthotic insoles generally are prescribed by a podiatrist (see page 29).

*Walkers' tips*

### KEEPING YOUR LACES TIED

**Choose carefully**
*Flat laces are less slippery than round ones (though round laces are easier to untie when they become wet).*

**Tuck them under**
*Double knot the bow and tuck all four ends under the crisscross lacing.*

**Tape them up**
*Run a piece of duct tape around the instep to hold the laces in place.*

**Keep them damp**
*Squirt a little water on the laces after they are tied. This will increase resistance and so prevent slipping.*

### When to replace your shoes

The outsoles of most walking shoes are made from tough carbon fiber, which can take plenty of hard knocks. It's the compressible midsoles, made of polyurethane or ethylene vinyl acetate (EVA) foam, that suffer most from wear and tear and so determine when you should replace your shoes. The function of the midsoles is to absorb shock. Each time your feet hit the ground, the midsoles are compressed, and with every compression, the midsoles lose a bit of their "spring." Podiatrists recommend that you replace your walking shoes about every 350 miles (560 km). So, if you're walking 2 miles (3.2 km) a day, five days a week, you'll need new shoes after about eight months. If you're overweight you may need to replace your shoes more frequently, as weight increases the pressure on the midsoles. Check also for obvious signs of wear—treads that have worn smooth, seams that have come apart or a worn padded lining.

### Which type of footwear should I choose?

It's best not to use your general sneakers or running shoes for walking. Many running shoes are not flexible enough and bend in the arch rather than at the ball of the foot. Some sneakers also have a fairly high heel— the heel should be no more than 1 in. (2.5 cm) higher than the rest of the sole. Avoid flared heel designs, because they prevent good heel-to-toe roll. Your choice of shoes or boots will depend on the terrain and the weather conditions in which you're likely to be walking. Brand names will vary, but these are the characteristics of the main types.

■ **Walking shoes** These are excellent for flat, smooth surfaces, such as you might find on city streets or in parks or malls. In contrast to tougher shoes designed more specifically for trails, walking shoes are ideal for walking at speed because the uppers do not go above the ankle, allowing maximum flex of the foot. The soles are often slightly rounded—if you place them on a flat surface and push the toes down, the heels rise. This gives a smooth heel-to-toe roll and also helps increase your stride length and speed. The midsoles will be slightly cushioned for maximum comfort on hard surfaces, and the uppers will probably be made from soft fabrics or leather.

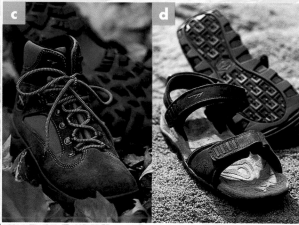

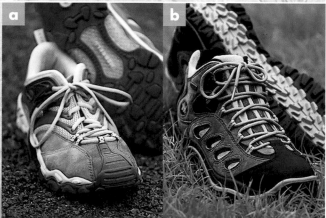

### Footwear for the terrain

**a Walking shoes** Provide flexibility and comfort on flat, smooth surfaces.

**b Trail shoes** Hard-wearing and with good grip for walking on trails.

**c Hiking boots** Sturdy support and protection for all types of rough terrain.

**d Sports sandals** For maximum breathability and good grip on all sorts of terrain.

- **Trail shoes or day hikers** Suitable for off-road walking, these are more robust and durable than urban walking shoes. Their slightly less flexible soles protect your feet from rough ground and their deeper treads offer better traction. Some come higher up the ankle to provide support. Look out for shoes with a Gore-Tex layer or made from leather to keep your feet dry.
- **Hiking boots** These are suitable for all hills, rough terrain and wet conditions. On challenging trails, particularly if you're carrying a heavy pack, you'll need a rigid boot with plenty of padding. To protect your ankles, choose boots that come high above the ankle and that have good torsional resistance (cannot be twisted easily from side to side). On more level ground, choose boots that come to midway up the ankle and that have less torsional resistance, giving you more flexibility. Hiking boots should have good traction on the outsole and a sturdy midsole. Choose boots with leather or synthetic uppers that are both waterproof and breathable.
- **Sports sandals** These are great for walking and hiking in hot weather. The new generation of sports sandals have good traction on the soles, similar to day hikers. They should have adjustable straps—usually three—to create a snug fit. When trying them on, make sure that there is at least 1 in. (2.5 cm) of space between your toes and the end of the shoe to prevent stubbing your toes.

## Socks

As with shoes and boots, you can buy socks designed for walking. For the good health of your feet, it's worth spending a little bit extra on socks suited to your needs. Also, you'll need to make sure you buy the correct size—too tight and they will restrict your toes, too loose and the "lumps" will irritate your feet.

### Consider the conditions

The most comfortable walking socks strike a balance between breathability and bulk. Although cotton sports socks are fine for shorter, on-road walks when warmth

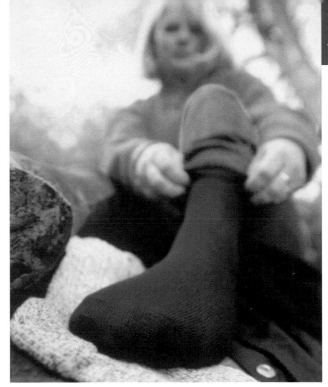

**A layer of warmth**
*Liner socks can be worn under wool or fleece socks to create a heat-retaining barrier for extra warmth.*

and wet are not factors, socks made with a "loop stitch" system, which improves both air circulation and cushioning, are the most effective way of achieving this balance. Wool-ragg socks are a particularly good option for winter, as they keep your feet warm even when it's wet. In summer, however, they can be uncomfortably hot. There are lots of synthetic materials and combinations that are perfect for year-round use— socks made with synthetics such as CoolMax keep you warm when it's cold and cool when it's hot. Also, don't neglect the sensibilities of your fellow walkers: Antimicrobial yarn, which is made with silver fiber, has effective antiodor properties, as well as giving socks a longer life span.

Some hikers use seamless, synthetic or silk liner socks under a pair of wool or fleece socks. In cold weather, these layers help keep feet warm by trapping air. For wet conditions, you can buy waterproof socks with a Gore-Tex or similar membrane sandwiched between the sock layers, though these are not quite as comfortable as regular socks.

## Clothing

There's no need for a wardrobe full of walking gear. If you choose items that can be worn in layers, then it's possible to get by on a limited number of year-round garments. Depending on the weather and your needs, the factors you should look for are: waterproofing, windproofing, breathability and freedom of movement.

### Jackets

Besides your footwear, a jacket is the most important garment you'll purchase. For comfort in all seasons, a combination of a waterproof outer jacket and an inner fleece is ideal. Use the outer jacket when it's wet and the inner when it's cold, or both when it's wet and

cold. Many good jackets also are made from breathable materials (see box, opposite), which is a good choice for optimum comfort. Although there are jackets with a detachable inner fleece available as one unit, you can buy the two items separately.

Although an outer layer will give you some protection from the wind, fleece jackets are great for walkers, as they are windproof as well as warm. Fleece is preferable to wool, as it is lightweight, dries very fast and retains heat when wet. Fleece comes in different densities, so check on the manufacturer's label that the one you buy is suitable for your needs: A denser fleece will give greater wind protection in difficult weather conditions, while a thinner fleece is sufficient in milder

## ANATOMY OF A JACKET

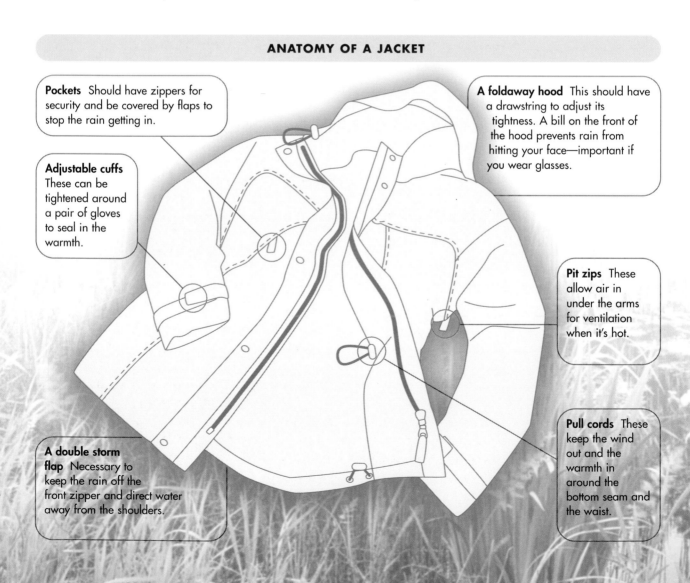

**Pockets** Should have zippers for security and be covered by flaps to stop the rain getting in.

**Adjustable cuffs** These can be tightened around a pair of gloves to seal in the warmth.

**A foldaway hood** This should have a drawstring to adjust its tightness. A bill on the front of the hood prevents rain from hitting your face—important if you wear glasses.

**Pit zips** These allow air in under the arms for ventilation when it's hot.

**Pull cords** These keep the wind out and the warmth in around the bottom seam and the waist.

**A double storm flap** Necessary to keep the rain off the front zipper and direct water away from the shoulders.

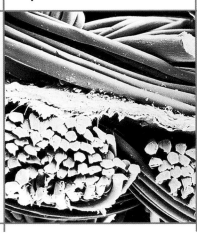

## BREATHABILITY AND WATERPROOFING | explained

Although removing layers is one way of keeping cool while exercising, it is a good idea to look for a jacket that is both waterproof and allows your body to breathe. Fabrics such as Gore-Tex, Sympatex, Hydroseal, Schoeller fabric or Dryskin are designed to do just this. Many of these work by having a coating on the back of the outer fabric covered with millions of tiny holes that are too small to let the rainwater in but large enough to let body vapor out. Some have a separate membrane also, which keeps the sweat away from your body until it can evaporate. Look out for jackets with pit zips, for extra breathability.

climates and will be lighter to wear and carry. Unisex jackets are common, but it's possible to buy men's or women's—men's will usually have longer arms.

### Tops

For all-weather walking, you'll need a base and an insulating layer. In cold climates, the air space between them maximizes warmth and comfort. T-shirts, long-sleeved tops or zip turtlenecks made from wicking polyesters and other synthetics are best for your base layer. Woolly looking knits, fleece sweaters or down vests provide great insulation. Remember that layers can always be removed if you get too hot.

In dry, warm weather, cotton shirts or T-shirts will keep you cool, while synthetic tops will wick away sweat from the skin. Look out for materials with ultraviolet (UV) protection to protect you from the sun.

### Pants

There are lots of fun pant designs out there with loads of pockets for storing gadgets. Zip-off legs give you shorts and pants all in one—great for changes in the weather. With materials, legs need similar protection to the upper body. In the summer, look out for cotton or synthetic pants that are light, breathable and offer UV protection. In winter, consider fleece or other synthetics that are warm, quick-drying and waterproof.

Waterproof and windproof overpants are useful for the cold and wet and are light enough to carry in your pack. Breathability is not as important with overpants, as they can be vented through pocket zippers. However, a zipped lower leg is essential for pulling pants on and off over footwear. Overpants should tighten at the cuff to prevent mud or snow getting in and be long enough to cover the tops of your shoes or boots, while still allowing plenty of movement.

Gaiters offer great protection to your lower legs and ankles when walking through rough undergrowth, snow or mud. They are waterproof and prevent water and mud from being splashed up the legs of your pants or from your foot to the opposite pant leg.

### Underwear

In all weather, you'll want to look for underwear made from comfortable and breathable fabrics. There are many garments available made from branded synthetics such as CoolMax, Ryovyl, Capilene or Dryflo, which wick away moisture from the skin to keep you dry. Some fabrics are also treated to resist the build up of odors and bacteria. Long- or short-sleeved T-shirts and long johns of silky synthetic fiber feel like a second skin and will keep you snug and warm in winter. You also can get briefs that are made with a wind-resistant panel for extra protection.

For women, a good sports bra is a must. Your everyday bra may not provide the support you need. Consider:

- **Fit** Make sure your sports bra fits snugly enough to control breast motion, but doesn't interfere with your breathing.
- **Support** Sports bras have either molded cups, which give firm support, or compressed cups, which flatten the breasts against the body. Larger-breasted women should opt for molded cups.
- **Fabric** Choose a blend of at least 50 percent cotton and a "breathable" material, such as Lycra mesh, to help evaporate sweat. Some are lined with wicking material under the breasts and arms.
- **Straps** Choose wide, non-stretch straps that won't dig into the skin and will provide maximum support. A wide "Y-back" panel will prevent straps slipping down the arms.

## Accessories

- **Gloves** Fleece is ideal when it's windy and wet, as it allows your palms and fingers to breathe and dries quickly. Keep the warmth in with an elasticized wrist or adjustable wrist fastening. More waterproof synthetics are available for wet conditions. Thermal liner gloves add to your warmth. Also consider mittens in very cold conditions, as they reduce the surface area from which heat can be lost.
- **Hats** Wide-brim hats give great protection from the sun and rain and many are designed to be "crushed" for easy storage. Safari-style hats with a wide piece of fabric attached at the rear protect the neck and can easily be folded up when not needed. Baseball caps are old standbys, giving shade and protecting the eyes from rain. If your neck is getting burned, wear a bandanna under your hat and let it hang down on your neck.
- **Scarves** A woolen scarf is great for warmth but not ideal in wet conditions, as wool takes a long time to dry and feels heavy. Fleece will dry quickly and still feel snug. For maximum warmth, fold your scarf in half lengthways and slip the open end through the loop made by the fold.

## Carrying your gear

Your choice of a fanny pack, day pack or backpack will be determined by the length of your walk and the amount of gear you wish to carry.

### Fanny packs and lumbar packs

These small bags are ideal for short walks, when you need just enough room for your lunch, water and waterproof jacket. Look for a comfortable hip belt that sits snugly on your waist. You may also want features such as water-bottle pockets, reflective taping or compression straps. Advantages of these are that you avoid getting a sweaty back, your arms are free to move and you don't have the room to carry needless stuff.

**Pack heavy items at the top**
*Keep the center of gravity in your pack level with or above your shoulders for better balance.*

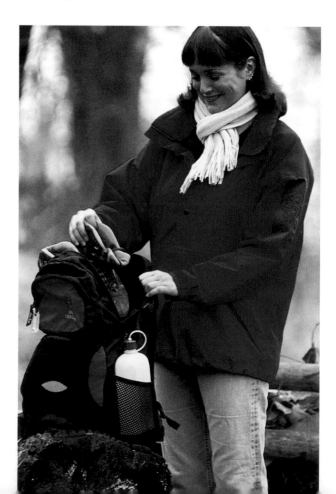

### Day packs

These are good if you're going to be walking for several hours and need to carry some water, snacks and perhaps a change of clothes. It's important to find a pack with straps that fit snugly over your shoulders. This will stop the pack from rubbing or moving too much as you walk. Some packs have meshing on the parts that rest against your back to keep it cool. A pack with plenty of pockets is also useful, particularly external pockets in which you can put items you need frequently. You also can buy packs with an internal drinking system (see page 132). Prices for day packs range from $30 to $100 depending on the quality of the stitching and materials and the number of features.

### Backpacks

If you're going on a trek where you'll be staying overnight, you'll probably need a backpack for all your clothing and equipment. Backpacks have either an external or internal frame. With an external frame the pack is not in direct contact with your back, so gives good ventilation. If you're walking in an area where balance is important, an internal frame is better as the pack's center of gravity is closer to your own. More expensive backpacks have shoulder-harness systems that you can adjust for a good fit. With all types of backpacks, foam-padded shoulder straps and a padded hip belt are important, since most of the weight will ride on your hips and shoulders.

## ANATOMY OF A DAY PACK

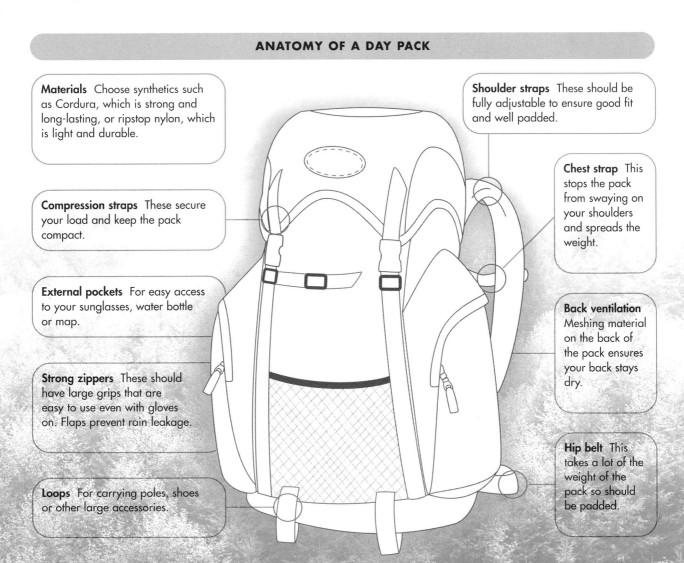

**Materials** Choose synthetics such as Cordura, which is strong and long-lasting, or ripstop nylon, which is light and durable.

**Compression straps** These secure your load and keep the pack compact.

**External pockets** For easy access to your sunglasses, water bottle or map.

**Strong zippers** These should have large grips that are easy to use even with gloves on. Flaps prevent rain leakage.

**Loops** For carrying poles, shoes or other large accessories.

**Shoulder straps** These should be fully adjustable to ensure good fit and well padded.

**Chest strap** This stops the pack from swaying on your shoulders and spreads the weight.

**Back ventilation** Meshing material on the back of the pack ensures your back stays dry.

**Hip belt** This takes a lot of the weight of the pack so should be padded.

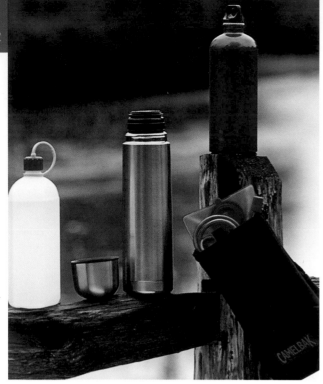

**Choosing a water container**
*Consider factors such as weight, price, capacity and usage when choosing between bottles, flasks and pouches.*

## Packing

Even with a large day pack it's important to pack properly. Your heaviest items, such as spare shoes, should go at the top of your pack and lighter items, such as a fleece, at the bottom. This will allow you to stand upright comfortably and prevent strain on your back. Always place items with hard or sharp edges away from the part of the pack that rests against your back or wrap them in clothing so they won't jab you.

## Bottles, pouches and flasks

If you're walking for more than 45 minutes, you shouldn't leave home without water. In the summer, even at a fairly sedate pace, the body can lose up to 4 pt (2.4 l) of water in just a few hours.

### Water bottles

There are two main types of water bottle: plastic or metal. A plastic or Nalgene bottle is simple, lightweight and virtually unbreakable. Carry it either in your pack or in a water-bottle holder that clips onto your belt. If it's in your pack, make sure it's easily accessible.

Plastic bottles can, however, leave an unpleasant aftertaste in your mouth. Metal bottles are good alternatives. Most are made from lightweight alloys, and, because metal is an excellent conductor, these bottles also keep your water cooler for longer than a plastic equivalent.

### Vacuum bottles

The insulating mechanisms in these bottles keep cold liquid cold and hot liquid hot. There are some great, compact, stainless-steel vacuum bottles available, but they often have the disadvantage of being quite heavy. On a chill winter's day, however, a steaming cup of coffee can make a flask well worth the extra weight.

### Water pouches and drinking systems

A water pouch is like a "tank," which you strap around your waist or carry on your back. A plastic pipe from the pouch reaches over your shoulder to your mouth. There are also plastic bladders available that fit in your pack and work in the same way. Some fanny packs have a large enough capacity to accommodate a water bladder, or come with one.

These carriers are ideal for long trips, because they have more capacity than ordinary water bottles, often up to 70 to 100 fl oz (1.8 to 2.5 l). They also encourage a more balanced intake of water—small, frequent sips, rather than the occasional large gulp, which can happen if your water bottle is stored in your day pack and you have to stop to drink it.

### Portable water filters

If you want fresh water as you walk, but don't want to carry it all, then a portable water filter is heaven-sent. These adapt to fit most types of water bottle or have a versatile plastic intake hose. Most filters remove a range of viruses, bacteria and protozoans. However, you should check that the filter you buy is appropriate for the area in which you're walking—the local water may contain microorganisms or heavy metals that your purifier cannot remove.

## Optional extras

The equipment mentioned so far includes the main items used for general walking. Here are some gadgets that might appeal to you for a particular type of walk.

### Maps

If you're leading a group or are walking in an unfamiliar area, a map is an extremely important piece of equipment. Even in an area you know well, a map can be useful to find new routes and gauge distances. In national parks, you will be able to get detailed maps at the park headquarters or visitor center, and these often include suggestions for routes. Alternatively, always try to get the largest scale map possible. Though you can buy maps that are laminated or made of heavy-duty paper, you might consider getting a map case to use when you're walking in bad weather. Soft, plastic cases are much better than hard cases, because you can fold them for easy access and storage.

### Map wheels

Also known as distance or mileage measures, these gadgets are used for calculating the distance you'll be going, which is particularly useful if you want to look at routes for a group walk. There are both electronic and mechanical versions available. To use, you simply run them over your route on a map, in either direction, and then read off the distance. You can read curved as well as straight lines and, with the electronic versions, you can calculate your expected time. Most models have a variety of built-in scales, so you can adjust the setting to match the scale of your map. However, don't rely on a map wheel for pinpoint accuracy—it's difficult to run them over a route perfectly, so they are best used as a general measure of distance.

### Heart-rate monitors

These used to be cumbersome contraptions, but modern versions are lightweight and hi-tech. Monitors fall into two camps: the photo-optic models and the electrocardio models, which tend to be more accurate (see page 144). Monitors range in price from about $25 to $250 or higher. Features to look out for include a stopwatch, a memory and a record of calories burned. Those at the top end might have a speaker that advises you if you need to pick up the pace. Go for one that has large, bold digits on the wristwatch so that you can read it easily when you're on the move.

---

### GLOBAL POSITIONING SYSTEMS | explained

The handheld global positioning system (GPS), which is about the size of a cell phone, has become a popular gadget with walkers. A GPS works by obtaining signals from satellites orbiting the earth, which it transfers to a dial. When you switch on, you get a grid reference, which you can compare against your map. Alternatively, you can program your GPS with maps of your area. Many models track the routes you have traveled and give you an average speed, as well as lots of other information such as altitude and sunset and sunrise times. These systems can be expensive, however, ranging from $150 to $300 or more. As they can also be inaccurate if you lose contact with the satellite, most walkers find a GPS works best as a complement to, not a replacement for, a compass.

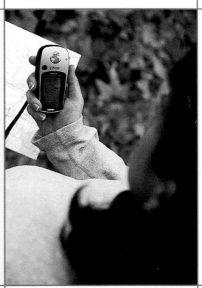

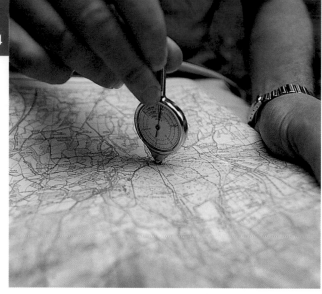

**Measuring a route**

*If you're a group leader, map wheels are good for evaluating distances and the time required for a route.*

## Pedometers and speedometers

These small, battery-operated devices measure the distance you walk, the steps you take, your average speed and even how many calories you're burning. This is based on your personal stride length, which you calculate when you first use your pedometer (see box, below). Costing about $15 to $85, the more expensive models have lots of "extras," such as a built-in radio, which you have to ask yourself if you really need. It is,

however, worth investing in a sensitive unit, as readings can sometimes be inaccurate and depend on the terrain you are walking on. Pedometers work best on flat terrain, with a steady stride. Your stride length alters when you ascend and descend steep hills so the reading won't be as accurate.

Much like pedometers, speedometers can measure your distance, speed and calories burned. However, these units tell how fast you're walking by means of a foot "pod" that attaches to your shoe.

## Trekking poles

Specifically designed for walkers, lightweight poles made of aluminum, fiberglass and titanium have become very popular in recent years. Their main advantage is that they add intensity to your walking, giving the muscles in your shoulders, back and chest a thorough workout, for maximum calorie-burning and toning. The poles also take a lot of pressure off your knees, especially during descents, and are wonderful if you have any other joint problems or mild arthritis. Though one pole can be a big help, they work most efficiently in pairs.

When choosing poles consider the following:
- **Adjustability (telescoping)** Most poles have two or three sections, so you can adjust your pole to a range of lengths—typically from 30 to 54 in.

## PROGRAMMING A PEDOMETER

First, measure a short distance, then walk it, counting your steps. Divide the distance by the number of steps. If the distance is 28 ft (8.5 m), for example, and the number of steps was 8, your stride length would be 3½ ft (1 m). Key this into your unit, clip it on and you're ready to go.

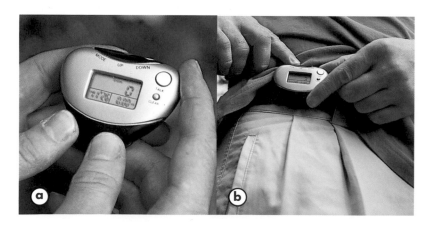

(76 to 137 cm) to suit your height. The adjustment range is particularly important if you're short or tall. A 6 ft 3 in. (1.91 m) person would need to adjust the pole to about 50 in. (1.27 m) for uphill walks, and even longer for downhill stretches, so that weight is transferred from the legs and lower back to the upper body. For this reason, avoid poles with a fixed length.

- **Weight** A lightweight but sturdy pole is ideal. Aluminum, aluminum alloy, titanium and carbon fiber are the best and most popular choices.
- **Antishock** Many poles have shock absorbers in their shafts to relieve stress on the hand, elbow and shoulder joints.
- **Handgrips and wrist straps** Angled ergonomic grips are designed to fit the shape of your hand. Grips are usually made of rubber or cork. The latter is particularly good if you want to avoid sweaty palms. Wrist straps are often lined with soft material for comfort and have a quick-release clip so you can adjust tightness without removing your gloves.
- **Packed length** Make sure the poles adjust down to a length that fits comfortably in or on the outside of your backpack—most can be reduced to about 25 to 30 in. (63 to 76 cm).
- **Tips and baskets** Spike metal tips of tungsten carbide are best for natural terrain, particularly rocky surfaces; rubber tips are used on the road. Some models combine the two, with a rubber foot that attaches to the metal part. Tips can accommodate various sizes of basket, which prevent the pole from sinking too far into the ground. For soft terrain choose wide baskets, around 3½ in. (9 cm) in diameter so your weight is spread over a larger surface area.
- **Price** Poles typically range from $60 to $150 per pair. At the top end models would include an antishock system, adjustable length, combined metal/rubber tip and padded wrist straps. Cheaper models may be of fixed length and not have as many comfort features.

## Walking sticks and canes

These popular accessories are great for local walks. Sticks and canes come with two different types of handles: the crook type, which is curved, and the support type, which is straight. It's the shaft, however, that will be taking the bulk of your weight, so make sure you use one that is sturdy enough to support you. These walking aids help propel you along in the same way as poles, so they may help you walk farther and faster. Look for a stick or cane with a rubber tip to prevent slipping, especially on wet ground.

**Walking safer**
*Over rough terrain and down hills it can be easy to lose your footing; poles are great at helping you maintain your balance.*

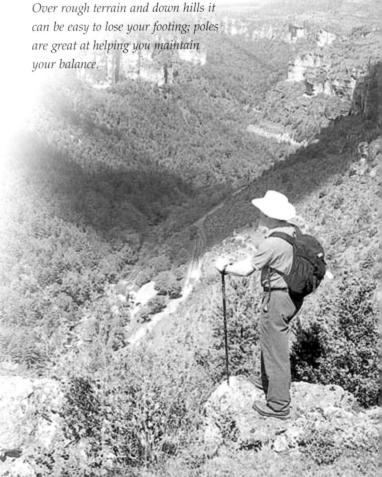

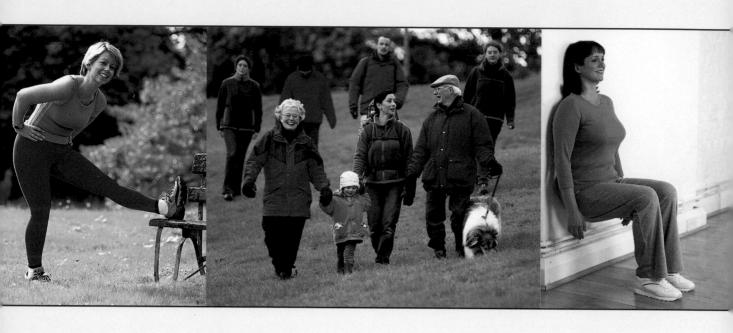

# WALKING
# PROGRAMS

*How to prepare for a program by testing your fitness and a selection of suggested programs to suit your needs and interests.*

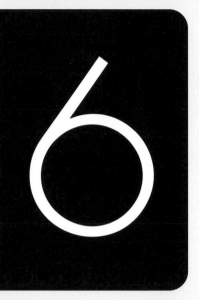

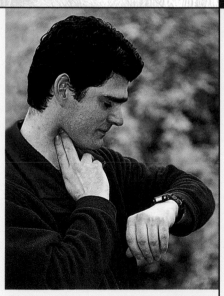

# SETTING YOUR **GOALS**

*One of the best ways to get motivated and stay motivated is to set goals. This section looks at choosing goals that are right for you and at how you make them work throughout your program.*

What inspired you to pick up this book? Did your doctor recommend you get more exercise? Or are you looking for a way to lose weight? Alternatively, someone may have given this book to you. If so, then you should bear something in mind—goals need to be personal. Your partner, friend, or relative may think you should keep your heart healthy, but what do you think? Even though you might agree that it's a good idea, lowering your blood pressure may not be the goal that motivates you into action; you might be more inspired by the thought of fitting into an old pair of jeans. Whatever your goal, make sure it relates to you personally or it will not provide the motivation to take up and maintain a walking program.

## *Realistic goals*

What do you want to get out of walking, and is it achievable? Walking a marathon by your next birthday may well be possible if you are fit already and have just had a birthday, but if you have only a month to train and you are out of shape, forget it. Similarly, if you're short and heavily built, accept that you'll never look like a supermodel. Walking can, however, give you a trimmer figure, a glowing complexion and a healthier heart. Be realistic about what walking can do for you, set your goals within your physical capabilities and you are more likely to succeed.

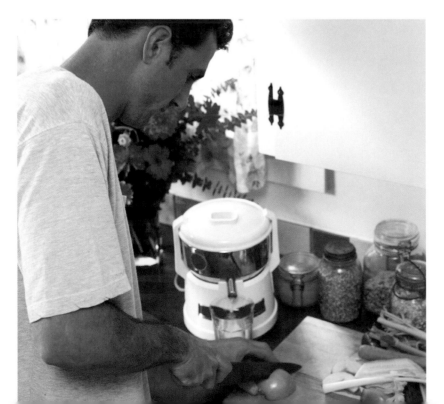

*"To travel hopefully is a better thing than to arrive, and the true success is to labor."*

ROBERT LOUIS STEVENSON

### Making lifestyle changes

*Your step-by-step goals need not be limited to walking. If you are walking to lose weight, factor a change in diet into your program. Plan your meals to include low-fat foods and set yourself weekly weight-loss targets.*

### Step-by-step goals

A general, long-term goal is not enough in itself. Setting smaller, more specific goals will let you know that you're on the right track and keep you motivated. If your goal is to improve your walking pace, and it initially takes you 20 minutes to walk a mile (1.6 km), try to reduce that time by 1 minute every two months. In addition, fine-tune your progress with smaller goals, such as trying to walk as fast as you can for at least 30 minutes every week. If you're trying to lose weight, losing 24 lbs (12 kg) is rather daunting; but setting a goal of 1 lb (0.5 g) a week means you'll have 25 weeks of victories. If you decide to track your progress, note down these goals in a diary or chart (see pages 182 to 183) and reward yourself for each step.

### Back-up goals

You have to accept that sometimes things just don't go according to plan. If you've been losing weight steadily for the past few weeks and one day you step on the scale to find that you've put on weight despite sticking to your regime, it can be extremely disheartening. But this isn't necessarily an indication that your program isn't working (see pages 158 to 161 for information on weight loss). By setting yourself additional goals, such as decreasing your waist measurement if you're trying to lose weight or lowering your heart rate if you're trying to improve your speed, you may find that while you haven't improved in one area, you've actually done really well in another.

At times, you may have to rethink your goals. If, for example, you trip and sprain your ankle, or your boss is away sick and you end up working 60-hour weeks, it's time for a back-up goal, which will keep you working toward your overall goal. You can try adjusting your methods: If, for example you're trying to lose weight and you suddenly find yourself unable to fit in a walk, try cutting down on your daily fat intake until you can return to walking. Or you could reassess your time frame: If the marathon is looming and you're not ready, find out about a half-marathon, instead.

*Walkers' tips*

## KEEPING YOUR GOAL IN SIGHT

### Write it down
*The simple act of committing your goal to paper will make it become a reality.*

### Display it
*Choose a prominent place to display your goal so that you'll see it on a daily basis. Stick it on your bathroom mirror, the fridge or on your car's dashboard.*

### Decide on your time frame
*Give yourself specific targets, such as increasing your speed by a percentage each month or losing 1 lb (0.5 kg) each week.*

### Record your progress
*Keep a note of how you're doing by jotting down distances and times in a notebook or making a chart that you fill in religiously.*

### Reward yourself
*When you reach a milestone, give yourself a treat. This can be as simple as a trip to the movies, lounging in the tub for an hour or pampering yourself with a massage. If you're attempting to lose weight, try to avoid using food as a reward.*

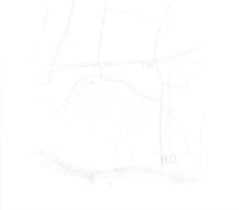

# PREPARE FOR YOUR PROGRAM

*You need to know your starting point to see how far you have to go and, later, what you've achieved. This section describes two basic fitness tests, as well as helping you understand intensity—how hard you should be working.*

The two main reasons that people take up exercise are to improve the condition of their hearts or to lose weight. The better you understand your fitness in these areas, the more focused your goals will be. Do the basic tests described here to assess your current level. The results will be useful when you're choosing a program. Subsequent tests will show your progress and, when you finish your program, provide a measure of your success. Photocopy the diary and chart on pages 182 to 183 to record your progress, or devise your own based on your goals.

Walking can, however, benefit more than just your heart and your weight. In addition to these tests, you may choose to assess your flexibility, strength and balance (see pages 178 to 181), or you may simply feel that fitness testing is not for you. In that case, just go ahead and enjoy walking—there is much more to overall health than physical fitness.

### Want to know more?

These home tests can provide you with basic indicators of fitness, but if you'd like to know more, seek professional advice and have a fitness test with a trained instructor. Your local gym should be able to help. It will have special equipment for testing fitness, giving more accurate readings than home tests.

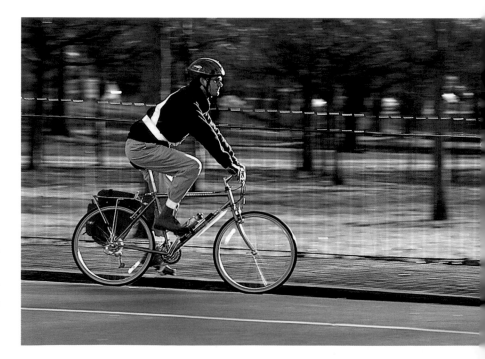

**Measuring a track**
*To perform the measured-track test, you'll need to find a course. Set your bicycle odometer to zero, then cycle the route for an accurate reading.*

## Testing your heart rate

Cardiovascular fitness is key for prolonging the length and quality of your life. It's also simple to test at home.

At rest, the average adult heart pumps 9 pt (5 l) of blood around the body every minute, and the typical adult has a resting heart rate of 72 beats per minute (bpm). The healthier and stronger your heart, the more blood it can pump. The difference between the resting heart rate of an unfit person and a fit person illustrates this: The heart of the unfit person beats at around 80 to 90 bpm, while the more fit heart only needs to beat at 50 to 60 bpm to fulfill the body's requirements. Some medicines also affect heart rate (see page 145).

For an approximate guide to your level of fitness, try taking your resting pulse rate using the technique described in the box, below. Make sure you've remained seated for at least 10 minutes before you take a reading—this gives your heart a chance to reach its resting rate. Note down your result, and then retest yourself after you've been walking for three months— you should see an improvement.

### SAFETY FIRST

The goal of exercise is to do yourself good, not to aggravate an existing problem. If you suffer from a heart condition or backache or answered "yes" to any of the questions on page 97, confirm with your doctor that it's safe for you to exercise. If you suffer from: pain or discomfort in your chest, neck or down your left arm; shortness of breath; dizziness; or nausea during or after your walk, stop and see your doctor.

### *Measured-track test*

With exercise, your muscles require more oxygen for fuel, and your heart will beat faster to meet the demand. To measure the efficiency of your exercising heart use the following test. Before you start, practice finding and taking your pulse (see box, below).

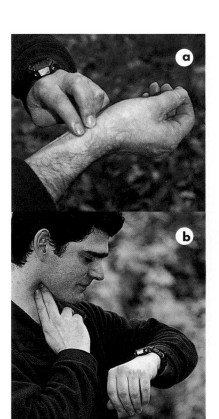

## TAKING YOUR PULSE

Find a watch with a second hand or seconds counter. Place your forefinger and middle finger on the inside of your wrist near the base of your thumb **a.** Press gently and you should feel your pulse. Do not use your thumb, because it is a pulse point as well. Using your watch, count the number of beats during 15 seconds. Multiply this number by four and you'll have your heart rate in bpm.

Alternatively, you can measure the pulse in your neck. It can be easier to locate and is stronger, particularly after exercise. Press gently with your forefinger and middle finger beneath your jawbone, slightly forward from your ear **b.** Don't press too hard, because it may affect your heart rate. Again, count the beats during 15 seconds and multiply by four to work out your heart rate.

For this test you'll need:

■ To be able to take your pulse;

■ A stopwatch or a watch with a second hand;

■ A 1-mile (1.6-km) course.

First, find your course. Ideally, it should be a flat, paved walkway or grassy surface. Measure a mile (1.6 km) as accurately as possible. You can do this by driving the course, by using a bicycle odometer or by looking on a large scale map. Alternatively, use the inside lane of an athletics track, which is a standard ¼ mile (400 m)—four times around this will give you your course.

Warm up for 5 to 10 minutes (see pages 36 to 37). If you've not exercised for a long time, you may need to warm up longer. When you are ready, start your stopwatch or note the time. Then walk the course as fast as possible without overexerting.

After completing the course check your time. Then immediately count your pulse for 15 seconds, and work out your heart rate in bpm. If you didn't finish the course, don't worry—as you improve your fitness you can work toward completing a mile. Now refer to the chart below. Look at the appropriate section for men or women, and find your age group and the heart rate most like yours. Read across and compare your time to the times listed in columns A and B.

▶ If your time is the same as or greater than the time in column A, you have a low fitness level.

▶ If your time is between the times in columns A and B, you have a moderate fitness level.

▶ If your time is the same as or less than the time in column B, you have a high fitness level.

### How it works

The measured-track test is a good guide to your aerobic fitness. It works by comparing your heart rate to the time it took you to complete the course. This is more accurate than simply timing yourself over a certain distance. If, for example, two 47-year-old men walk the same 1-mile (1.6-km) course in 17 minutes, but at the end of the walk the first man's heart rate is 160 bpm while the second man's is 130 bpm, the second man is more fit.

Make a note of your result and time. Redo the test every three months to see how walking is improving your fitness—more often than this and you may not see any significant change. If you complete the course in the same time, you should notice that your heart rate has decreased. Alternatively, you may complete the course with the same heart rate, but with a faster time. These both mean that your body is getting more fit.

### HOW FIT IS YOUR HEART?

| | Age | 20 to 29 | | 30 to 39 | | 40 to 49 | | 50 to 59 | | 60+ | |
|---|---|---|---|---|---|---|---|---|---|---|---|
| | | A | B | A | B | A | B | A | B | A | B |
| | 110 | 20:57 | 19:08 | 19:46 | 17:52 | 19:15 | 17:20 | 18:40 | 17:04 | 18:00 | 16:36 |
| | 120 | 20:27 | 18:38 | 19:18 | 17:24 | 18:45 | 16:50 | 18:12 | 16:36 | 17:30 | 16:06 |
| MEN / Heart rate (bpm) | 130 | 20:00 | 18:12 | 18:48 | 16:54 | 18:18 | 16:24 | 17:42 | 16:06 | 17:01 | 15:37 |
| | 140 | 19:30 | 17:42 | 18:18 | 16:24 | 17:48 | 15:54 | 17:18 | 15:36 | 16:31 | 15:09 |
| | 150 | 19:00 | 17:12 | 17:48 | 15:54 | 17:18 | 15:24 | 16:48 | 15:06 | 16:02 | 14:39 |
| | 160 | 18:30 | 16:42 | 17:18 | 15:24 | 16:48 | 14:54 | 16:18 | 14:36 | 15:32 | 14:12 |
| | 170 | 18:00 | 16:12 | 16:54 | 14:55 | 16:18 | 14:25 | 15:48 | 14:06 | 15:04 | 13:42 |

## Understanding intensity

If you walk farther, more frequently or for longer periods of time, you'll benefit more from your walking. But if you want to really boost your fitness levels you'll need to walk more intensively—by walking faster, using your arms or walking on different terrains (see pages 44 to 53). Intensity can be measured, and the ability to compare one walk to the next is particularly useful if and when you do a walking program.

In technical terms, "exercise intensity" refers to how much oxygen your working muscles use during your workout: The harder you work, the more fuel your muscles require; the more fuel they require, the more oxygen they need to burn fat. Because there is a direct relation between the amount of oxygen used by your body and how fast your heart is beating, exercise intensity is usually measured by looking at your heart rate. However, measuring intensity need not be all that technical. Although you can use a heart-rate monitor (see page 144), you can also take your pulse manually or use your judgment to assess your effort level. These checks are important when walking, because if your intensity levels are too low, you'll see little benefit from your exercise, and if they're too high, you'll tire quickly and won't get the best out of your walking.

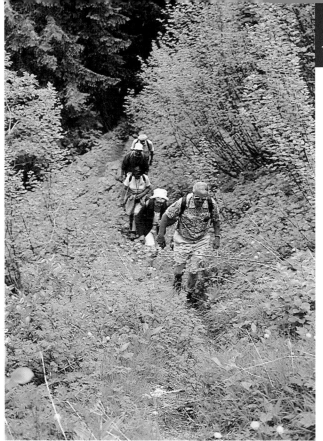

**Adding intensity**
*Walking uphill increases the resistance against which your leg muscles move. Varied landscapes also add interest to your walks.*

| Heart rate (bpm) | Age | 20 to 29 | | 30 to 39 | | 40 to 49 | | 50 to 59 | | 60+ | | |
|---|---|---|---|---|---|---|---|---|---|---|---|---|
| | | A | B | A | B | A | B | A | B | A | B | |
| | 110 | 19:36 | 17:06 | 18:21 | 15:54 | 18:05 | 15:38 | 17:49 | 15:22 | 17:55 | 15:33 | WOMEN |
| | 120 | 19:10 | 16:36 | 17:52 | 15:24 | 17:36 | 15:09 | 17:20 | 14:53 | 17:24 | 15:04 | |
| | 130 | 18:35 | 16:06 | 17:22 | 14:54 | 17:07 | 14:41 | 16:51 | 14:24 | 16:57 | 14:36 | |
| | 140 | 18:06 | 15:36 | 16:54 | 14:30 | 16:38 | 14:12 | 16:22 | 13:51 | 16:28 | 14:07 | |
| | 150 | 17:36 | 15:10 | 16:26 | 14:00 | 16:09 | 13:42 | 15:53 | 13:26 | 15:59 | 13:39 | |
| | 160 | 17:09 | 14:42 | 15:58 | 13:30 | 15:42 | 13:15 | 15:26 | 12:59 | 15:30 | 13:10 | |
| | 170 | 16:39 | 14:12 | 15:28 | 13:01 | 15:12 | 12:45 | 14:56 | 12:30 | 15:04 | 12:42 | |

**Source: The American Heart Association**

## HEART-RATE MONITORS | explained

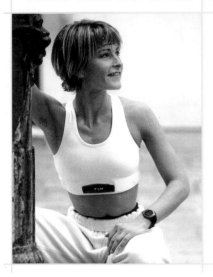

An alternative to taking your pulse is the heart-rate monitor, which measures your heart rate electronically. There are two main types available. Photo-optic monitors clip on to your earlobe or fingertip and shine infrared light through your skin to measure the amount of blood being pumped into your blood vessels. This information is transferred to a digital screen. Unfortunately, changes in daylight and movement of the sensor can give a skewed reading. Electrocardio monitors have a chest strap with a transmitter and watchlike receiver, and measure the electrical activity of your heart with a radio signal. They are usually more accurate than photo-optic monitors. As some women find it difficult to keep a chest strap in place, some transmitters can be fitted into special sports bras.

### The effects of working harder

Sometimes people put off exercising because they don't like the thought of "being sweaty and out of breath." If your lifestyle is not particularly active, you may not be used to feeling your heart beating faster and your breathing becoming quicker, and you might find the physical changes quite uncomfortable. But it's exactly this faster, stronger heartbeat and the quicker, deeper breathing that will lead you to better fitness. As long as you're not overdoing it, this is what you should aim for.

### Monitoring your heart rate

The speed at which your heart beats depends on your level of fitness and your age—generally, the older you get, the slower your maximum heart rate. Fitness professionals use this knowledge to set guidelines on how hard your heart should be working during exercise. These are based on percentages of the average maximum heart rate for your age.

To calculate your maximum heart rate in beats per minute (bpm), subtract your age from 220. For example, the average maximum heart rate of a 40-year-old person is 180 bpm. As this is only an average, your actual maximum heart rate may be 10 bpm either side of this figure.

Next, work out the intensity you should be working at—sometimes referred to as your "training zone"—which should be between 60 and 80 percent of your maximum heart rate. To calculate these percentages, simply multiply your maximum heart rate by 0.6 and then by 0.8. For the 40-year-old, this works out to be between 108 bpm and 144 bpm. As you walk, take your pulse regularly or use a heart-rate monitor (see box, above) to check that you are working within your "training zone."

### HEART RATE DURING EXERCISE

| Age | Max. heart rate | Heart training zone |
|---|---|---|
| 25 | 195 | 117 to 156 |
| 30 | 190 | 114 to 152 |
| 35 | 185 | 111 to 148 |
| 40 | 180 | 108 to 144 |
| 45 | 175 | 105 to 140 |
| 50 | 170 | 102 to 136 |
| 55 | 165 | 99 to 132 |
| 60 | 160 | 96 to 128 |
| 65 | 155 | 93 to 124 |
| 70 | 150 | 90 to 120 |

Highly trained individuals sometimes work at more than 80 percent of their maximum heart rates, but 60 to 80 percent is sufficient for most people to improve and maintain fitness. If you're unfit, start by exercising at the bottom end of your range. If you suffer from a heart condition or if you can't work at 60 percent of your maximum heart rate for very long, don't worry; try to work at about 50 percent and gradually build up. You will be surprised how quickly you improve.

Some medications can affect your heart rate, particularly those that relate to your heart or blood pressure. If you're taking anything that might affect your heart rate, such as beta blockers to control angina or blood pressure, it's better to use talk tests or the rate of perceived exertion method (see below) to monitor how hard you're working.

## THE BORG SCALE

| Numerical rating | Rating in words | Description |
| --- | --- | --- |
| 6, 7, 8 | Extremely light | You are barely moving, maybe standing to do the dishes |
| 9, 10 | Very light | Walking around the house or strolling |
| 11, 12 | Light | Walking at a slow pace |
| 13, 14 | Moderate | Walking at a moderate pace |
| 15, 16 | Hard | Walking at a brisk pace |
| 17, 18 | Very hard | Walking at a fast pace |
| 19 | Extremely hard | Walking at a brisk pace up a hill |

### Talk tests

A simple way of judging approximately how hard you're working on your walk is the talk test. All you need to do is talk as you walk and consider how difficult you find this. You don't need anyone else to be there, you can talk to yourself, as long as it's out loud.

▶ If your breathing is low and level, and you could easily shout out loud, you're not working hard enough and should speed up.

▶ If you can carry on a conversation without gasping for breath, you're doing a low-intensity walk.

▶ If you can say a few phrases, though you may be slightly breathless, you're doing a moderate-to-high-intensity walk.

▶ If it's quite difficult to speak and you're feeling quite breathless, you're working at a high intensity. You may want to limit the time you walk at this level.

▶ If it is very difficult to talk and you're very breathless, then you may be working too hard. Slow down a little or stop and march in place until you're able to talk more easily, and then resume your walk.

### Your rate of perceived exertion

Another very simple way of measuring intensity, which you may find easier than measuring your heart rate, is using a rate of perceived exertion (RPE) scale. These scales are widely used by exercise experts to determine exercise intensity. They work by encouraging you to listen to your body when you walk. Rather than using your pulse or a monitor to calculate your heart-rate measurements, you rate your effort level by how hard you think you're working.

One such RPE scale is the Borg Scale—named after the scientist who invented it—which uses a system of numbers and words to describe intensity. In studies, it has been shown that people exercising at 70 percent of their maximum heart rate consistently describe this intensity as "moderate" or between 13 and 14 on the Borg Scale. So, for health purposes, working between 12 and 15 on the Borg Scale will put you right where you should be—walking fast without overexerting. For most people, this corresponds to a moderate-to-brisk walking pace. But remember that this is a personal scale, so you may need to walk at a slower or faster pace than someone else to feel that you're working at the right intensity. Use the chart above to determine your intensity levels. Make a note of the various walking paces that correspond to the ratings in your scale, and refer to this chart as you build up your effort levels. The effort levels in the Borg Scale are used in some of the programs later in this chapter.

## Testing your body weight and shape

One of the major reasons people take up walking is to lose weight, whether for the good of their health or just to look more toned and feel better about themselves. But "losing weight" is about much more than just the needle on the scales. Although you're unlikely to look like a bodybuilder after a walking program, you'll develop and build muscles in your legs, torso and arms. Muscle is heavier than fat and this sometimes masks weight loss on the scales. So it's important to have more than one goal and use more than one of these tests. An easy way to judge your body shape and size is to keep two pairs of "reference" slacks—one pair you used to fit into and the ones you're currently wearing—try both pairs on every month to see how you're doing.

### Weighing yourself

A steady drop on the scales can be very encouraging to your walking. However, it's important to remember that your weight can change by as much as 5 lbs (2.25 kg) each day, and that it will vary at different times of the day. To make your comparisons as accurate as possible, weigh yourself while naked, at the same time each day. Either weigh yourself every day or once a week and stick to that pattern. If you have a Chinese meal one night and then weigh yourself in the morning, you may be shocked to see just how much weight you gained. This is because Chinese food is very high in salt, which causes your body to retain water. Some schools of thought suggest that weighing yourself every day will help you understand these fluctuations and not become too despondent if you happen to have a "heavy" day. Other people feel that weighing yourself once a week is sufficient and more encouraging, because it shows a more dramatic change in weight each time.

### Working out your waist-to-hip ratio

The difference in size between your waist and your hips can be used to determine your body shape, which, in turn, can be used as a guide to how much fat you're carrying. This test is easy to do, all you need is a tape measure and a calculator. Measure your waist at its narrowest point. Then measure your hips at their widest point. Finally, divide your waist measurement by your hip measurement. For example, a person with a waist measurement of 31 in. and a hip measurement of 35 in. would do the following: $31 \div 35 = 0.88$.

Studies have shown that men who have a waist-to-hip ratio greater than 1 and women who have a waist-to-hip ratio greater than 0.85 have a higher risk of developing heart disease. Aim to keep your waist-to-hip ratio below these figures.

### Your body mass index

If ever you've visited your doctor with concerns about your weight, he or she may have worked out your body mass index (BMI). This is a mathematical calculation that relates your body weight to your height. It does have its limitations, however, as your BMI says nothing about your body composition—how much of your weight consists of muscle and fat. For this reason, top

### CALCULATING YOUR BODY MASS INDEX

| Height (ft in.) | Weight (lbs) | | | | | | | | |
|---|---|---|---|---|---|---|---|---|---|
| | 100 | 105 | 110 | 115 | 120 | 125 | 130 | 135 | 140 |
| 5'0" | 20 | 21 | 21 | 22 | 23 | 24 | 25 | 26 | 27 |
| 5'1" | 19 | 20 | 21 | 22 | 23 | 24 | 25 | 26 | 26 |
| 5'2" | 18 | 19 | 20 | 21 | 22 | 23 | 24 | 25 | 26 |
| 5'3" | 18 | 19 | 19 | 20 | 21 | 22 | 23 | 24 | 25 |
| 5'4" | 17 | 18 | 19 | 20 | 21 | 21 | 22 | 23 | 24 |
| 5'5" | 17 | 17 | 18 | 19 | 20 | 21 | 22 | 22 | 23 |
| 5'6" | 16 | 17 | 18 | 19 | 19 | 20 | 21 | 22 | 23 |
| 5'7" | 16 | 16 | 17 | 18 | 19 | 20 | 20 | 21 | 22 |
| 5'8" | 15 | 16 | 17 | 17 | 18 | 19 | 20 | 21 | 21 |
| 5'9" | 15 | 16 | 16 | 17 | 18 | 18 | 19 | 20 | 21 |
| 5'10" | 14 | 15 | 16 | 17 | 17 | 18 | 19 | 19 | 20 |
| 5'11" | 14 | 15 | 15 | 16 | 17 | 17 | 18 | 19 | 20 |
| 6'0" | 14 | 14 | 15 | 16 | 16 | 17 | 18 | 18 | 19 |
| 6'1" | 13 | 14 | 15 | 15 | 16 | 16 | 17 | 18 | 18 |
| 6'2" | 13 | 13 | 14 | 15 | 15 | 16 | 17 | 17 | 18 |
| 6'3" | 12 | 13 | 14 | 14 | 15 | 16 | 16 | 17 | 17 |
| 6'4" | 12 | 13 | 13 | 14 | 15 | 15 | 16 | 16 | 17 |

athletes could be labeled "overweight," because muscle weighs more than fat, and they carry more muscle than average for their heights. But, in general, your BMI can provide a useful indication of whether you need to gain or lose weight.

Weigh yourself in the morning without clothes. If you don't know your height in bare feet check it first. Find your weight and height on the chart below and read along to where the two meet. For example, if you're 5 ft 6 in. (168 cm) and weigh 123 lbs (56 kg), your BMI is between 19 and 20—a healthy weight for your height.

▶ If your BMI is 18.5 or below, you're underweight.

▶ If your BMI is between 18.5 and 25, you're a healthy weight for your height.

▶ If your BMI is between 25 and 30, you're overweight, and should reduce it to below 25.

▶ If your BMI is more than 30, you're clinically obese and you should seek the help of your doctor or a nutritionist to lose weight.

## Calculating your fat percentage

Testing your body composition—how much of your body is made up of fat—is a very good guide to fitness. However, you do need to visit a gym or buy a special device to measure your body fat. Some devices (priced around $45 to $250) look like digital bathroom scales and work by sending a small electrical current through your body. The amount of electrical resistance shows your fat percentage, because electricity doesn't flow as well through fat as it does through other tissues. There are also body-fat calipers available (around $45 to $70 or more), which are used to pinch folds of skin at various points on your body to get an overall estimate.

The "optimal" fat percentages, according to health professionals, are between 12 and 20 percent for men and between 16 and 26 percent for women. Carrying a little bit of extra fat is not a problem if you're otherwise fit and healthy, but if you reduce your fat percentage by even a few points you'll find you look and feel a whole lot better.

| 145 | 150 | 155 | 160 | 165 | 170 | 175 | 180 | 185 | 190 | 195 | 200 | 205 | 210 | 215 | 220 | 225 | 230 | 235 | 240 | 245 | 250 | Height (ft in.) |
|---|---|---|---|---|---|---|---|---|---|---|---|---|---|---|---|---|---|---|---|---|---|---|
| 28 | 29 | 30 | 31 | 32 | 33 | 34 | 35 | 36 | 37 | 38 | 39 | 40 | 41 | 42 | 43 | 44 | 45 | 46 | 47 | 48 | 49 | 5'0" |
| 27 | 28 | 29 | 30 | 31 | 32 | 33 | 34 | 35 | 36 | 37 | 38 | 39 | 40 | 41 | 42 | 43 | 43 | 44 | 45 | 46 | 47 | 5'1" |
| 27 | 27 | 28 | 29 | 30 | 31 | 32 | 33 | 34 | 35 | 36 | 37 | 37 | 38 | 39 | 40 | 41 | 42 | 43 | 44 | 45 | 46 | 5'2" |
| 26 | 27 | 27 | 28 | 29 | 30 | 31 | 32 | 33 | 34 | 35 | 35 | 36 | 37 | 38 | 39 | 40 | 41 | 42 | 43 | 43 | 44 | 5'3" |
| 25 | 26 | 27 | 27 | 28 | 29 | 30 | 31 | 32 | 33 | 33 | 34 | 35 | 36 | 37 | 38 | 39 | 39 | 40 | 41 | 42 | 43 | 5'4" |
| 24 | 25 | 26 | 27 | 27 | 28 | 29 | 30 | 31 | 32 | 32 | 33 | 34 | 35 | 36 | 37 | 37 | 38 | 39 | 40 | 41 | 42 | 5'5" |
| 23 | 24 | 25 | 26 | 27 | 27 | 28 | 29 | 30 | 31 | 31 | 32 | 33 | 34 | 35 | 36 | 36 | 37 | 38 | 39 | 40 | 40 | 5'6" |
| 23 | 23 | 24 | 25 | 26 | 27 | 27 | 28 | 29 | 30 | 31 | 31 | 32 | 33 | 34 | 34 | 35 | 36 | 37 | 38 | 38 | 39 | 5'7" |
| 22 | 23 | 24 | 24 | 25 | 26 | 27 | 27 | 28 | 29 | 30 | 30 | 31 | 32 | 33 | 33 | 34 | 35 | 36 | 36 | 37 | 38 | 5'8" |
| 21 | 22 | 23 | 24 | 24 | 25 | 26 | 27 | 27 | 28 | 29 | 30 | 30 | 31 | 32 | 32 | 33 | 34 | 35 | 35 | 36 | 37 | 5'9" |
| 21 | 22 | 22 | 23 | 24 | 24 | 25 | 26 | 27 | 27 | 28 | 29 | 29 | 30 | 31 | 32 | 32 | 33 | 34 | 34 | 35 | 36 | 5'10" |
| 20 | 21 | 22 | 22 | 23 | 24 | 24 | 25 | 26 | 26 | 27 | 28 | 29 | 29 | 30 | 31 | 31 | 32 | 33 | 33 | 34 | 35 | 5'11" |
| 20 | 20 | 21 | 22 | 22 | 23 | 24 | 24 | 25 | 26 | 26 | 27 | 28 | 28 | 29 | 30 | 31 | 31 | 32 | 33 | 33 | 34 | 6'0" |
| 19 | 20 | 20 | 21 | 22 | 22 | 23 | 24 | 24 | 25 | 26 | 26 | 27 | 28 | 28 | 29 | 30 | 30 | 31 | 32 | 32 | 33 | 6'1" |
| 19 | 19 | 20 | 21 | 21 | 22 | 22 | 23 | 24 | 24 | 25 | 26 | 26 | 27 | 28 | 28 | 29 | 30 | 30 | 31 | 31 | 32 | 6'2" |
| 18 | 19 | 19 | 20 | 21 | 21 | 22 | 22 | 23 | 24 | 24 | 25 | 26 | 26 | 27 | 27 | 28 | 29 | 29 | 30 | 31 | 31 | 6'3" |
| 18 | 18 | 19 | 19 | 20 | 21 | 21 | 22 | 23 | 23 | 24 | 24 | 25 | 26 | 26 | 27 | 27 | 28 | 29 | 29 | 30 | 30 | 6'4" |

# CHOOSING A PROGRAM

*Walking is limitless: You can do it wherever and whenever you want. To improve your physical fitness, you need to build up your walking over time. This section introduces a range of walking programs.*

The walking programs in this book are designed as a guide to structuring your walking over a period of time so that you're increasing the frequency, duration, length and intensity of your walks. The best way to get the most from walking is to walk every day. This is why all the programs incorporate a Daily Dose of walking, even if it's just for 10 minutes (see box, opposite). In addition to this, walking should become a habit and part of your lifestyle.

To free up time for a workout or an aerobics class, some people end up driving to the gym rather than walking. This is why the overriding message of these programs and, in fact, this book is to walk whenever and wherever possible. If you're following a program, this "lifestyle walking" can count toward your daily and weekly targets.

## Choosing a program

When you're deciding which program to work with, there are two things to consider: your goals and your level of physical fitness. It may be obvious which of the programs most closely matches your goals, and that's a

good place to start. But if you want to improve your fitness overall, then you might prefer to start with one of the general programs: Beginner's, Intermediate or Advanced. In this case, you should perform one or more of the fitness tests on pages 140 to 147. Check the list at the start of each program to see which one most suits you. Even if your physical fitness is good but you're new to walking, you may need to start at a lower level until your body adapts to it. Very few other forms of exercise involve the same movements that fast walking requires, and you may need time to perfect your technique. When you complete a program, try moving on to the next.

### Devising your own program

If you do want to follow a program, but find none of these suitable, then create your own, using these as a guide. Sit down with a pen and paper and make a timetable. Plan your walking according to your level of fitness, building up slowly through the weeks and recording your progress. Work out exactly when you can fit in a period of walking for each day of the week—you may find it easier to stick to your program if you walk at the same time each day and it becomes part of your routine. If you really cannot get out walking one day try to identify another day when you can double your walking time.

If you're trying to improve your heart health, for example, first test your cardiovascular fitness (see pages 141 to 142), and then using your current level as a starting point, build target intensity levels (see pages 144 to 145) into your program.

### THE LATEST EVIDENCE

A study by K.R. Westerterp, published in *Nature*, demonstrated that people who incorporate exercise into their daily activities—walking to work rather than driving, or taking the stairs rather than the elevator—expend more energy overall than people who exercise only at specific times.

Remember, however, that it will take time to build your fitness. If you're struggling to meet your targets, or if you feel you could do more, think again. You may need to revise your program. You'll need at least three months to see major changes.

## How to use the programs

Once you've selected a suitable program, following it is simple. Each one is designed to be carried out over a period of 10 to 12 weeks and includes suggested walking amounts and intensities for each week. The way that intensity is measured—in percentages of your maximum heart rate or rate of perceived exertion (RPE)—is described on pages 143 to 145. If you miss days or weeks of your program, pick up where you left off. Remember, too, that back-up goals can be good if outside pressures cause you to stop your program.

> **Daily Dose**
> For each program there is a recommended Daily Dose, which appears in a box like this. If you have trouble completing the length and duration of the walks in the full program, try to walk at least this amount—it will bring benefits.

### Choosing a set route

Many of the programs require you to walk a set route. The route you choose will vary according to the health goals you have. However, all routes should be easily accessible from your home and be in areas in which you enjoy walking. A large-scale local map can help you choose routes and measure distances.

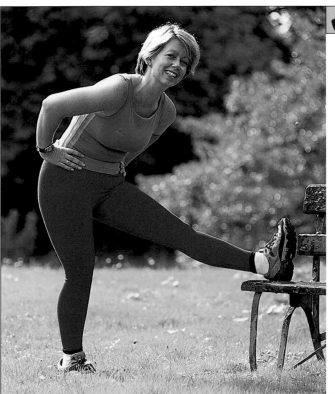

## ✓ AM I READY FOR A PROGRAM?

❑ **Walking technique** Check your technique before you start (see pages 24 to 33). It will help you walk farther and faster and avoid injuries.

❑ **Health questionnaire** If you answered "yes" to any of the questions on page 97, see your doctor before taking up walking.

❑ **Fitness tests** These do more than just help you decide where to start, use them to record your progress and achievements.

❑ **Warm up and cool down** On walks of 20 minutes or more you'll need to include a warm-up and cool-down. Check you know how on pages 34 to 43.

❑ **Goals** Set yourself targets, both long and short term. For advice, see pages 138 to 139.

# BEGINNER'S PROGRAM

**Use this program if:**

▶ You haven't had any exercise at all for the past three months

▶ You're not used to walking regularly, having done less than 30 minutes a week for the past three months

▶ You're overweight, have a BMI of more than 25, or a waist-to-hip ratio of 1 or more if you're male, or 0.85 or more if you're female

▶ You're unable to walk a mile (1.6 km) or can't walk this distance in less than 18 minutes

▶ You have a medical condition mentioned on page 97, but your doctor has said that you can take up walking

This program aims to introduce you to walking regularly and to take you to a level at which you can walk for 30 minutes at a moderate-to-brisk pace at least five times a week. By picking up this book, you've already taken the first step toward achieving that goal. In just three months, you should see significant improvement and will be ready to move on to the intermediate program.

The important things to remember over the following weeks are: Build up your walking gradually, and stick to a pace and distance that are comfortable for you. Don't worry if you're not quite as fit as you expected, you'll soon see improvements. You should be able to carry on a conversation easily while you're walking and should not experience any pain, although you might feel slightly uncomfortable if you're new to walking. If the discomfort persists after

## Week 1

**Day 1** Walk around your local streets for around 20 minutes. You can rest after 10 minutes or split your walk into two 10-minute sessions, if you prefer. Try to walk at a "light-to-moderate" level (RPE of 11 to 13), or at about 55 to 65 percent of your maximum heart rate.

**Day 2** Repeat the walk you did on Day 1. Think about posture and technique. Don't worry too much about speed.

**Day 3** If you're tired, do just your **Daily Dose**. If you found Days 1 and 2 manageable, explore your neighborhood for 30 minutes.

**Day 4** Planning day. Consider the areas you've explored so far and, using a map, devise a set route that you can do at any time. Ideally it should be between 1 and 2 miles

(1.6 to 3 km) in length, with good, even surfaces that will be walkable in all weathers. If possible, make it a route which starts from your front door or place of work. Try to incorporate some green space and quiet streets.

**Day 5** Try out your set route, timing yourself as you go. Walk at an RPE of 12 to 13, or at about 55 to 65 percent of your maximum heart rate. Note your time.

**Day 6** Just do your **Daily Dose**.

**Day 7** Walk your set route at a "light-to-moderate" level and time yourself. If you have a heart-rate monitor, aim for 55 to 60 percent of your maximum heart rate.

## Week 2

Try to walk your **Daily Dose** every day this week.

In addition, walk your set route at least twice at a "light-to-moderate" level (RPE of 12 to 15), or at about 60 to 75 percent of your maximum heart rate. Note your time, and try to reduce it, even by a few seconds.

Fit in one further walk lasting 40 minutes to 1 hour during this week at a "light-to-moderate" level. Try to make it different from your set route.

**Daily Dose**

Walk for 10 minutes every day at a moderate pace. Walk wherever you choose—outside, in your garden, or in the local mall.

**POSITIVE THINKING**

► These first few months are a chance for your body to get used to walking. Stick to your own pace—only you know when you're ready to progress.

► This is your introduction to walking, so enjoy it. Smile at people who pass, listen to the birds or admire the flowers in a window box.

► Remind yourself regularly of your goals. Each walk is bringing you closer to what you want to achieve.

► Use these early walks for exploring the area in which you live. There may be a street that you've previously overlooked or a park you haven't visited.

► Test your fitness after the first three months. If you've stuck to your program, you're bound to see results.

you stop walking or if you experience pain, then you're pushing yourself too hard and you need to slow down to a more comfortable pace. Try measuring the intensity of your walks using one of the techniques on pages 143 to 145. Also, refer to pages 24 to 33 if you need a reminder of the correct technique and posture.

## Weeks 3 to 5

At a minimum, walk your **Daily Dose** every day.

Walk your set route at least once a week. Aim to improve your time by a minute by Week 5. While you're doing your set route, spend 5 to 10 minutes walking at a "moderate-to-hard" level (RPE of 14 to 15), or at about 70 to 75 percent of your maximum heart rate. This should make you slightly out of breath.

Take two longer walks during these three weeks of between 45 minutes and 1 hour. Try to walk at a slightly out-of-breath pace for at least 20 minutes of the walk.

## Weeks 6 to 11

Continue to walk your **Daily Dose** every day.

Also, walk your set route twice a week, timing yourself each time and keep to your improved pace. Start looking at ways to extend your set route for future weeks.

Each week complete at least one additional longer walk lasting around an hour. During this session and your set walk, try to make yourself become slightly out of breath for at least 20 minutes of the time, working at a "moderate-to-hard" level.

## Weeks 12+

Walking should now be an integral part of your lifestyle. You should be able to walk 1 mile (1.6 km) without becoming exhausted and in less than 18 minutes. If you find this a struggle, then continue with the program for Weeks 6 to 12 until you find it more comfortable.

Now look at ways of increasing the intensity of your walking—using your arms more, and/or incorporating hills (for further suggestions, see pages 70 to 85 ). Gradually lengthen the time you walk and the distance you cover, trying to walk at a "moderate-to-hard" level for periods of 15 to 25 minutes in any one walk.

# INTERMEDIATE PROGRAM

## Use this program if:

▶ You've been exercising regularly for at least three months, but are looking for a change

▶ You're used to walking and are capable of 30 minutes a day at least five times a week

▶ You can walk a mile (1.6 km) in 16 minutes

▶ You're of average weight, have a BMI of 18 to 25 or a waist-to-hip ratio of less than 1 if you're male or less than 0.85 if you're female

▶ You answered "no" to all of the questions in the questionnaire on page 97 or your doctor has approved this level of exercise

This program will provide you with a framework for lifelong, sustainable health and fitness. If you already enjoy walking but feel you're not getting enough from your current level of activity, then this program can help you to walk more quickly and effectively.

This intermediate level of walking is one that you can adopt at any time in your life and that conveys all the health benefits you need to keep you fit and happy. The amount and intensity of walking involved meets the minimum weekly levels of physical activity recommended by many health professionals and organizations, including the U.S. surgeon general (see opposite). The program will push you hard enough to make you feel fantastic and make walking a part of your daily routine. Although you might feel slight discomfort as you get used to the correct walking technique, this should not last; if it persists or

## Week 1

**Day 1** Find a set route that you can access regularly and easily. It should be mostly level, but may include a few hills, and should take you between 30 and 45 minutes to walk at a moderate-to-brisk pace. Check on a map that your route is at least 2 to 3 miles (3.2 to 4.8 km). If the route includes hills, it can be slightly shorter.

**Day 2** Walk your set route quickly but without overexerting. Time yourself and note it down.

**Day 3** Walk your **Daily Dose** at a moderate-to-brisk pace.

**Day 4** Go for a longer walk of 45 minutes to an hour. Try to find a new route and, wherever possible, seek out green spaces. Walk at a "moderate" level (RPE of 13 to 14), or at about 65 to 70 percent of

your maximum heart rate, for at least 20 to 30 minutes of the time.

**Day 5** Take a rest today and use the time to think of ways that you can incorporate walking into your daily routine.

**Day 6** Walk your set route again, but don't worry so much about your pace or time. Focus on posture and technique. If you feel any discomfort, refer to pages 24 to 33.

**Day 7** If you're tired, walk your **Daily Dose** in two periods of 10 minutes. Look at your reflection in store windows and check that you're walking tall. If you feel up to it, take a longer walk.

## Week 2

Walk your **Daily Dose** and try to walk at a brisk pace for part of it.

Replace one or two of your **Daily Dose** walks with longer walks of about 45 minutes to 1 hour. These should incorporate 5-to-10-minute periods at a "hard" level (RPE of 15 to 16), or at about 75 to 80 percent of your maximum heart rate.

Use all the opportunities you have to be active, such as walking to the stores or to work and walking the kids to school.

> **Daily Dose**
> Walk for at least 30 minutes five days a week. You can split this into two periods of 15 minutes, but make sure you're walking at a level that you find is moderate to hard.

## RECOMMENDED LEVELS OF ACTIVITY

According to a report from the U. S. surgeon general on "Physical Acitivity and Health," more than 60 percent of adults in the United States do not get the recommended levels of weekly physical exercise. The report found that physical exercise need not to be strenuous, but that moderate activity should be undertaken on most or all days of the week to achieve significant health benefits. Such activity includes walking 2 miles (3.2 km) in 30 minutes or stairwalking for 15 minutes.

if you start to experience any pain during your walking, slow down, you may be pushing too hard. Stick to a pace and distance that's comfortable, and if you can't keep up with all of the recommendations, at the very least, do your **Daily Dose**.

## Weeks 3 to 5

Do your **Daily Dose** on most days that you don't do a longer walk and work at a "moderate" level.

Walk your set route once a week at a moderate-to-brisk pace. Time yourself and try to cut 1 minute off your initial time by Week 5.

Also, do one long route of 45 minutes to an hour once a week, working at a "hard" level. Alternatively, walk for 30 minutes in an area with a hill. Try to maintain a moderate-to-brisk pace as you go uphill, watching your posture and technique.

## Weeks 6 to 12

Continue with your **Daily Dose** and try to walk at a "hard" level for at least 10 minutes.

Also, walk your set route at least once a week, timing yourself. See how you've improved.

Try to do two long walks each week, lasting between 45 minutes and an hour. Walk at a brisk pace for most of the time, working at a "hard" level (RPE of 15 to 16).

As an alternative to the two long walks, include hills on at least two of your shorter weekly walks and maintain a brisk pace.

## Week 12+

Your **Daily Dose** should now be part of your everyday life. There may be some days when you don't manage to walk, and you can, in some part, make up for this by walking longer or farther the next day. But it's better to walk whenever you can. If possible, leave the car at home for trips of less than 1 mile (1.6 km). On longer walks you should work at a brisk pace, at the "hard" level, for at least 20 minutes of the time.

You can remain at this level as long as you want to, since it will provide you with the activity you need to maintain your health. If you want to challenge yourself further, you're ready for the advanced walking program (see pages 154 to 155).

# **ADVANCED** PROGRAM

## Use this program if:

▶ You've been walking regularly for three months or more and have not experienced an injury

▶ You're able to walk 1 mile (1.6 km) in less than 15 minutes and a gentle hill without being winded

▶ You're of average body weight and you have a BMI of between 18 and 25, or a waist-to-hip ratio of less than 1 if you're male, or less than 0.85 if you're female

▶ You're free of medical conditions mentioned in the questionnaire on page 97 or your doctor allows you to step up the pace

▶ You're active and want to supplement your exercise with a low-impact alternative to running

Do you want a challenge? This is a program for those who walk regularly but want to improve their speed and fitness levels. Though daily walking is a feature, the more demanding walks each week will improve your fitness and keep you in shape.

Research has shown that walking can bring about the sort of fitness benefits that were previously thought to be associated only with running and other aerobic sports. An advanced program will add intensity to your walking by incorporating increased speed and distance and inclines into your walks. You'll also improve your upper-body fitness and strength by increasing the amount you use your arms while walking. You can achieve this by focusing on arm control (see page 27) and by using poles as you walk (see page 50). You may want to think about investing in a heart-rate monitor to help you track your progress

## Week 1

**Day 1** Find a set route measuring 3.5 to 5 miles (5.6 to 8 km) which is easily accessible. It should include slight hills, be paved and without major roads. You should be able to walk it in 40 minutes to 1 hour.

**Day 2** Time yourself as you walk your route as fast as you comfortably can. You should still be able to talk, but be working at a "moderate-to-hard" level (RPE of 14 to 16), or at about 70 to 80 percent of your maximum heart rate for most of the walk. Try to maintain your pace when walking hills.

**Day 3** Walk your **Daily Dose** at a brisk pace. Watch your posture and technique.

**Day 4** Walk for 45 to 60 minutes at a moderate-to-brisk pace. Make sure you find some green spaces to

walk in—being close to nature will relax your mind and your body.

**Day 5** Walk your set route. Once you've warmed up, include a few 5-minute periods of faster walking at a "hard-to-very hard" level (RPE of 15 to 17). You may feel discomfort in your shins, but the short periods will help your body get used to the new demands on it.

**Day 6** Walk your **Daily Dose**, even if it's only at a moderate pace.

**Day 7** Take an hour-long walk today in a scenic spot and focus on your form. Are you walking tall? Are your shoulders relaxed? Are your abdominal muscles pulled in?

## Week 2

If nothing else, continue with your **Daily Dose**. If you're unable to walk at all on any particular day, replace it with some other exercise or activity.

In addition, walk your set route twice this week, timing yourself and trying to shed a few seconds off your original time.

Include one long walk of up to 1 hour. Walk at a "moderate-to-hard" level for the duration of your walk. In this long walk include at least two 5-to-10-minute periods of fast walking, increasing your speed with shorter, quicker steps and pumping your arms so that even on flat ground you're working hard.

> **Daily Dose**
>
> If nothing else, walk for at least 30 minutes every day. This can be broken down into two periods of 15 minutes, but you should try to walk at a "hard" level whenever possible.

more easily. Also, consider having your fitness tested by a professional.

Before you begin this program, it's vital that your technique is as near perfect as possible, to make sure that you're not putting yourself at risk of injury. If you're satisfied that your technique is good, then you're ready to start kicking things up a gear.

## BREAKING THE SPEED BARRIER

Despite repeated efforts, you may reach a point at which you don't seem to be able to reduce your time on your set route. Don't take this as a sign that your fitness isn't improving. When you're exercising, your brain and nerves "fire" impulses to your working muscles, causing them to contract. The speed at which these impulses are fired determines how fast your legs move. Your nervous system needs training in the same way as your body. Start with shorter periods of fast walking and gradually extend the time you spend at high speed. Your brain and nerves will gradually adapt and be able to send messages to your working muscles faster.

## Weeks 3 to 5

Walk your **Daily Dose** every day; this will ensure that walking becomes a habit. Already you may find that you're walking much more in your daily life and reaching for the car keys a lot less.

Try to do three further hard walks a week. This can consist of doing your set route at a brisk pace or going on long walks of an hour or more, which include 10-minute periods of fast walking. Continue pumping your arms; this will help your legs go faster. You can build up your upper-body strength further by incorporating some wall presses into the cool-down section of your walk (see page 180). You should, by now, be feeling much more fit.

## Weeks 6 to 11

At a minimum, continue with your **Daily Dose**.

On top of this, do at least three hard walks a week lasting 20 minutes or more. Remember you can walk for shorter distances at a faster pace or longer distances at a slower pace to achieve similar results. Make one of these walks your set route and time yourself. You should find that your speed has improved and you may have shaved a minute or more off your starting time.

Walk whenever and wherever you can. Continue with wall presses and consider other weight training— speak to a gym instructor.

## Weeks 12+

Continue with the **Daily Dose**; it should now be a part of your day's routine, as important to you as brushing your teeth.

Keep up the hard walking for an hour or more on three days a week. For at least 20 minutes of these walks you should be pushing yourself so that you're quite out of breath. Work at a "hard-to-very hard" level (RPE of 15 to 17), or at about 75 to 80 percent of your maximum heart rate.

Start exploring new routes with more challenging hills, and incorporate new techniques into your walks, such as the walk-run technique, or using poles or resistance (see pages 44 to 53).

# WALKING FOR A **HEALTHY HEART**

**Use this program if:**

▶ You're not generally active but are concerned about keeping your heart healthy

▶ You're unable to walk a mile (1.6 km) in less than 20 minutes or can't walk a mile

▶ You're overweight, have a BMI of more than 25, or a waist-to-hip ratio of 1 or more if you're male, or 0.85 or more if you're female

▶ You have a heart condition—a previous heart attack, angina or high blood pressure—and your doctor has recommended that you increase your levels of physical activity

With cardiovascular disease being the number one cause of death in the United States today, and lack of physical exercise being a major risk factor for heart disease, walking can be an excellent way of protecting yourself. This program will show you how to introduce walking to your everyday life so that you can develop a strong and healthy heart.

Your heart is a muscle, and this means it needs to be exercised regularly to keep it strong and healthy. Even leisurely walking done for 30 minutes a day can bring benefits, and the ultimate aim of this program is to bring you up to, or approaching, that level of walking. This will improve the condition of your heart and keep the blood vessels clean and open. In addition to this, walking can help to reduce other factors that contribute to heart disease, such as high blood pressure, excess weight and stress.

## Week 1

If you've had some recent heart problems then check with your doctor to see whether you can start to exercise.

If you can't manage your **Daily Dose**, try to walk for 10 minutes at least three days this week. Choose a different route for each walk to find the one that suits you best.

Choose a few flat routes close to your home. Go as far as is comfortable, take it slowly and with as many stops as you need. Work at an "extremely light-to-very light" level (RPE of 8 to 10), or at about 40 to 50 percent of your maximum heart rate. Don't overexert yourself this week; the most important thing is that you've started.

## Week 2

Start improving the function of your heart by walking at least 5 days a week. This will be your **Daily Dose** of 10 minutes a day. Find a steady, comfortable speed. Work at a "very light-to-light" level (RPE of 9 to 11), or at about 45 to 55 percent of your maximum heart rate.

These walks will not only increase your life expectancy, but also give you more energy, as your heart begins to release more oxygen. Try new routes and enjoy being outside. Don't let the weather keep you indoors. Wind and rain can be invigorating.

## Week 3

Continue with your **Daily Dose** at least 5 days this week.

Concentrate on the lengths of your walks. Replace one of your **Daily Dose** walks with a longer walk of 30 minutes or replace two **Daily Dose** walks with walks of 15 minutes. The pace can be as slow as you like. These walks will help you keep down your blood-sugar levels and reduce your cholesterol level. These, in turn, help keep your arteries open and your blood flowing freely.

If you've suffered a heart attack or currently suffer from angina or high blood pressure, then see Walking with a Heart Condition (pages 98 to 99) for further information and consult your doctor before starting an exercise program. During the early weeks of the program, focus on building up the time you spend walking, rather than the intensity. Try not to walk at more than 65 percent of your maximum heart rate, always remembering the phrase "walk fast without overexertion." You should be working at a "very light-to-moderate" level (RPE of 9 to 14) according to the Borg Scale on page 145.

> **Daily Dose**
>
> If you don't manage any of the longer walks each week, take 10-minute walks five days a week. This is enough to get your heart muscle working. Five short walks are better than two longer walks.

## Week 4

Continue with your **Daily Dose**.

Also, try to go for one longer walk lasting 30 minutes or three walks lasting 15 minutes. Begin to increase your pace slightly to get the heart muscle pumping and improve your aerobic fitness. Over the last 3 weeks your heart has been gradually warming up. Now you need to give it a gentle workout. You should be working at a "light" level (RPE of 11 to 12), or at about 55 to 60 percent of your maximum heart rate. This will make the heart stronger and able to work with less effort, leaving you with more energy.

## Weeks 5 to 10

Try now to build your **Daily Dose** into your everyday routine, whether it replaces a short errand you normally drive, or becomes a morning stroll.

**Week 5** Plan out a set route. Study a local map and, using your knowledge of the area, plot a route 1 to 2 miles (1.6 to 3.2 km) long. Make sure it's easily accessible, and preferably away from heavy traffic. Time yourself as you walk the route. Remember not to push too hard; you should be working at a "very light-to-moderate" level (RPE of 9 to 13), or at between 45 and 65 percent of your maximum heart rate. Repeat this set route at least once a week as well as doing your **Daily Dose**.

**Weeks 5 to 7** Build up your walking so that you're going out for a total of 30 minutes a day for at least three days a week as well as doing your **Daily Dose**. If necessary, divide the 30 minutes into two 15-minute walks.

**Weeks 8 to 10** Build up your walking again so that you're going out for 30 minutes a day for at least 5 days a week.

**Week 10** Walk your set route and time yourself again. You should notice an increase in your speed without any extra effort. This is proof that your heart is becoming stronger and more efficient.

# WALKING FOR **WEIGHT LOSS**

*If you've been struggling with your weight for years, a good diet and exercise can do wonders. Unlike many sports, walking can become so much a part of your routine that you don't even know you're exercising.*

The number-one reason that people gain weight is because they take in more energy—measured in calories—in the form of food than they expend in the form of exercise. The way to lose weight is just as simple: Eat less and exercise.

People often give up vigorous exercise, such as jogging or working out at the gym, because they don't actually like it or because the activity is too physically demanding. Walking, however, is something that anyone can do safely and happily, and, as it is so easy to keep up, is an exercise that helps with the long-term weight loss that can be so difficult for so many people.

## How exercise helps

In theory, a calorie eaten is equal to a calorie used (see box, opposite), so cutting down on food should bring about the same weight-loss results as increased exercise. In reality, however, this equation proves less clear-cut. Time and time again dieting alone has been shown to be less effective in keeping off the weight than a good diet and exercise.

### Boosting your metabolism

Every day—even if you stay in bed—your body uses a certain amount of calories: to circulate the blood, for

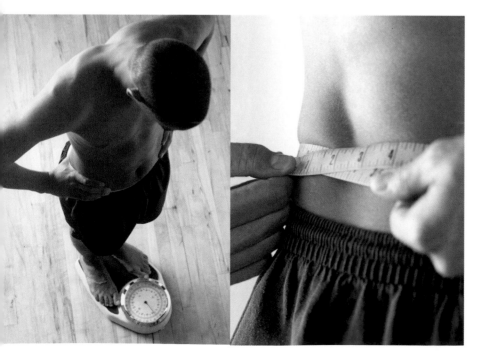

### Varied measures

*Although weighing yourself can be an encouraging way of monitoring your weight, using a range of checks, such as your body mass index or waist-to-hip ratio, will provide more accurate results (see pages 146 to 147).*

digesting food, to grow cells and for all other bodily processes. The amount of calories this requires is called your basal metabolic rate (BMR), and it is separate from the energy you need for physical activities such as walking. Each person's BMR is different, and it depends on your sex, weight, stature and, in particular, how much fat you're carrying compared with muscle, as muscle tissue burns calories even while you are at rest. The more fit you are, and the more muscles you have, the more calories you burn just to stay alive.

As you walk, you're not only burning fat, but also building muscles, so your body is burning calories long after your walk has finished. And once the weight is lost, walking regularly will ensure that it stays off.

### Achieving your ideal weight

If you've measured your body weight and composition (see pages 146 to 147), you'll have determined whether you fall into the "normal" ranges for your body mass index (BMI) and/or your waist-to-hip ratio. Although these measurements are used by health organizations to give ideal body weights and figures, they may not reflect your aspirations for your weight. You may feel that they are too lenient, and you know that you're happier if you weigh a little less; or you may feel that they are too stringent, and you can't believe that you'll ever meet those targets. Don't let charts and figures put you off. If you prefer not to measure yourself in this way, make your goal simply to be more fit and more healthy. The weight will slowly, but surely, drop off.

Even if your weight is still well within the guidelines, you should keep an eye on it. As we get older, our bodies slow down and expend less energy. Someone over 40 who takes less than 30 minutes of moderate exercise a week, may gain on average about 2 lbs (0.9 kg) a year. Just consuming an extra 75 calories a day—one chocolate cookie—beyond the energy you expend would lead to an annual weight gain of almost 8 lbs (3.6 kg) a year. However, a daily 30-minute walk can burn 120 calories or more.

---

## THE ENERGY BALANCE | explained

The equation that explains why we gain or lose weight is very simple: If you consume the same amount of energy as you use each day, then, under normal circumstances, your weight should remain constant. When there are imbalances in this scale, you'll start to see changes in your weight: If your calorie intake is more than your energy output, you'll gain weight; and if your calorie intake is less than your energy output, you'll lose weight.

You can make the scales go in your favor by eating fewer calories, increasing your exercise level, or by doing a combination of the two. A healthy diet alongside increased exercise is by far the best option; not only does attacking the issue from both sides require you to sacrifice less food, but it also will bring the healthiest and most long-lasting results.

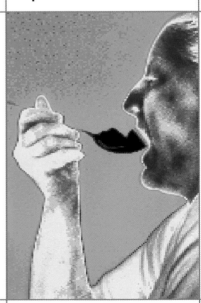

# PROGRAM FOR **WEIGHT LOSS**

**Use this program if:**

▶ You're overweight, have a BMI of more than 25, or a waist-to-hip ratio of more than 1 if you're male or more than 0.85 if you're female

▶ You're unable to walk 1 mile (1.6 km) in less than 18 minutes

▶ You're looking to lose weight in the short term and keep it off in the long term

▶ You've tried other forms of exercise but you don't enjoy them and/or can't find the time

▶ You want to reduce your risks of heart disease and stroke by losing excess fat and strengthening your heart

Walking is ideal for losing weight; it's gentle enough for anyone, but brings enough fat-burning benefits to make a difference. Also, walking allows you to go at your own pace so that you build up your fitness gradually. This program offers a realistic, safe and effective solution to the weight-loss battle.

The program will bring benefits on its own, but if you want to really get the most from weight-loss walking you need to pay attention to your diet at the same time. Try to reduce your intake of fats and refined sugars and starches, such as white bread, french fries, cookies, cakes, ice cream, candy and soft drinks. Instead eat plenty of fruit and vegetables, white meat, fish and unrefined carbohydrates, such as cereals and whole-grain bread, pasta and rice. These foods give you the energy you need for exercise but won't make you put on as much weight (see pages

## Week 1

**Day 1** Although walking at any pace will burn calories, you'll burn more calories the faster you walk. Start walking at a "moderate" pace.

**Day 2** Walk for at least 10 minutes today, thinking about your posture. Concentrate on pulling in your abdomen and walking tall; this will instantly make you look slimmer.

**Day 3** Walk for 20 minutes at a moderate-to-brisk pace. Walk for an additional 10 minutes at another time of the day—whether you visit a friend or go out on your lunch break.

**Day 4** Before you go out, think of a route that you'll be able to follow on any day of the year and that ideally starts at your front door. It should be 1 to 2 miles (1.6 km to 3.2 km) long. Try it out; it should take you no more than 40 minutes.

This is your set route. You can always fall back on it if you don't want to venture farther afield.

**Day 5** Walk your set route and time yourself. Walk as fast as you can without overexerting.

**Day 6** Walk for two periods of 15 minutes at a moderate pace.

**Day 7** Go for a longer walk today of up to 1 hour, and try to walk at a moderate-to-brisk pace for at least 20 minutes of the time. Work at a "light-to-moderate" level (RPE of 12 to 13), or at about 60 to 65 percent of your maximum heart rate.

## Week 2

Continue with your **Daily Dose**. Whenever possible, try to increase your walking time to 45 minutes.

Also, do one longer walk of up to one hour, including 20 minutes at a "moderate-to-brisk" level. During this time work at 60 to 70 percent of your maximum heart rate, with an RPE of 12 to 14.

If you have a day when you really can't fit in time for a walk, try to reduce your calorie intake to compensate for the lack of activity.

90 to 91). As they boost your intake of fiber, they fill you up for longer and reduce your urge to snack.

The more walking you do, the more quickly you'll lose weight. But don't rush it; the secret to losing weight and keeping it off is to lose weight gradually, at a rate of about 1 to 2 lbs (0.5 to 1 kg) a week.

## THE VALUE OF WALKING

A 150-lbs (68-kg) person walking on level ground will expend the amounts of energy shown below. The calories burned are even higher if you're walking up hills, with poles or on a sandy beach.

| Walking speed | Average calories burned in 1 hour |
|---|---|
| Slow, around 2 mph (3.2 km/h) | **240** |
| Moderate, around 3 mph (4.8 km/h) | **280** |
| Brisk, around 4 mph (6.4 km/h) | **420** |
| Fast, around 4.5 mph (7.2 km/h) | **500** |

### Daily Dose

Walk 30 minutes a day at a moderate pace. This burns about 110 to 170 extra calories, so try to do this every day of the week.

## Weeks 3 to 5

Walk your **Daily Dose** every day of this week, but make it last 45 minutes on at least four of these days, broken down into 15-minute periods if necessary. Work at a "moderate" level for the duration of the walk (RPE of 13 to 14) or at about 65 to 70 percent of your maximum heart rate.

Replace one of your **Daily Dose** walks with your set route at least once a week. Aim to cut your time, even by a few seconds.

You may start to notice the effects of all this exercise on your body shape and size during these weeks. This should encourage you to keep going. Check that you're still meeting your goals.

## Weeks 6 to 11

Continue with your **Daily Dose**, walking for 45 minutes at least four days a week. If you're following a diet, this is a point at which weight loss might start to hit a rut. Add hills and use your arms so that you burn off even more calories. At 3.5 mph (5.5 km/h) on hills your energy expenditure is 400 to 500 calories per hour (see page 48).

Again, replace one of your **Daily Dose** walks with your set route at least once a week, trying to improve your time with each walk.

Take one longer walk every week and explore the area around you for new routes to increase variety and keep you motivated.

## Weeks 12⁺

Your **Daily Dose** should now be an integral part of your life. Keep it that way and the weight will stay off.

In addition, look for longer walks and inspiration. Find new places to explore and friends to walk with—consider joining a walking group.

If you've stuck to your healthy eating and regular walking, the results will now be obvious. You'll look slimmer and more toned. If you weighed yourself or worked out your BMI or waist-to-hip ratio before you started, check them again. If you haven't achieved as much as you'd hoped, you may just need more time, so stick with the program.

# WALKING AWAY FROM A **BAD BACK**

**Use this program if:**

► Your work requires you to spend prolonged periods at a computer screen or behind the wheel of your car

► You experience stiffness in your back first thing in the morning

► You often feel tension and soreness in your back, neck or shoulders

► You're recovering from a mild back injury

► You've been advised against more strenuous forms of activity, such as weight training, because of the stress this will put on your back

Most of us will suffer back pain at some time in our lives. Often this is no more than a minor irritation, but sometimes it can be a considerable problem that affects our performance at work and our family life. This program has been designed to help relieve back stiffness and pain, and to gradually increase your back's mobility and strength.

One reason backache may be so common is because of changing lifestyles. Our ancestors evolved to run through forests hunting for food, and now we only hunt for food on the supermarket shelves. This, combined with our tendency to spend long periods driving or sitting in front of a computer screen, can lead to recurrent back problems.

Physical therapists, physicians, orthopedists, chiropractors and osteopaths all recommend walking to bring relief from back pain, as it is an effective but

## Week 1

**Day 1** Get started. Walk a distance you can manage without too much effort, such as from your front door to a neighbor's house or to the store. Repeat this short walk at least once today.

**Day 2** Walk the same route again. Try to walk early in the day when stiffness and pain are often at their worst. If your pain increases as you walk, try to keep going slowly until it improves. It's important to stretch out your muscles after every walk (see pages 40 to 43). To get the maximum benefit try to hold each stretch for at least 30 seconds. If, however, any of the stretches cause you pain, discontinue them and seek medical advice.

**Day 3** Rest today. Look over any local maps you have and plan other routes you may want to walk.

**Day 4** Get out twice and walk for at least 10 minutes each time. Concentrate on posture and foot placement (see pages 26 to 27).

**Day 5** Walk your **Daily Dose** today. This is a week for evaluating your body's limitations and possibilities. If you experience discomfort and it becomes severe, consult your doctor.

**Day 6** Go out three times today, even if it's only for 10 minutes each time. Increase the distance of one of the walks.

**Day 7** Walk your **Daily Dose**. Walk tall and keep good posture in mind. Check on it often by looking at your reflection in store windows, if possible.

## Weeks 2 to 3

If nothing else, walk your **Daily Dose**. The key is to walk briefly and often, strengthening your back muscles and keeping your back warm and mobile. Remember your stretches, particularly those that stretch your hamstrings.

Try to double your **Daily Dose** in these weeks, building up to two walks a day lasting 10 to 15 minutes each.

> **Daily Dose**
> Seize any opportunity to walk during the day, even if it's simply a walk around the room. Try to walk for at least 10 to 15 minutes every day.

low-risk form of exercise. If your backache is related to weight gain, then walking also can help ease pain by helping you lose pounds. Back pain is often the result of poor posture, so pay particular attention to your technique as you walk (see pages 26 to 29). Properly fitting shoes (see page 29) are also essential to ensure correct alignment of the spine.

## SAFETY FIRST

You should always make sure that at the onset of any particular back problem you visit your doctor. It's highly unlikely you'll be told walking is not a good idea or that it's likely to increase your pain, but you do need to identify the root of your problem. Don't worry if walking causes initial discomfort, because this should settle quickly. If discomfort worsens or is prolonged, however, then go back to your doctor.

## Weeks 4 to 6

Build up your **Daily Dose** so that you walk for 20 to 30 minutes a day, five days a week, or do two walks of 15 minutes each day. Gradually increase the distance and pace of your walks.

In addition to your daily walking, walk around the room or up and down the stairs for a few minutes at least once every couple of hours.

Avoid sitting for long periods of time and think about your posture. Walking with your shoulders rounded or your upper body leaning forward are surefire ways to back pain. If you complement your outdoor walking with a treadmill session, this will help you focus on your form.

## Weeks 7 to 9

As your back pain improves, walk farther and faster. Try to walk for 30 minutes every day in these weeks. Don't worry if your progress seems slow at first—everyone is different and so is every back.

Vary the route to add interest. Wherever possible try to give your walk a practical purpose by walking your errands rather than driving, and take advantage of every opportunity to walk.

## Weeks 10⁺

Continue with the program for weeks 7 to 9. As walking becomes a part of your daily routine, so should stretching. Stretch out your back, shoulders, neck and chest to relieve tension. Relax in a warm bath if your muscles are feeling sore after a walk.

By now you should be experiencing relief from your back pain, and you should also be feeling the benefits of the weight that you've lost as a result of your walking program.

# WALKING WITH **OSTEOPOROSIS**

**Use this program if:**

▶ You've been diagnosed with osteoporosis and your doctor has suggested that you increase your level of exercise

▶ You've a history of osteoporosis in your family

▶ You've gone through the menopause

▶ Your BMI is less than 18.5 or you've dieted a lot during your lifetime

▶ You don't eat a balanced diet or foods rich in calcium and vitamin D

▶ You take, or have taken in the past, medication that weakens the skeleton, such as corticosteroids to treat rheumatoid arthritis, Crohn's disease or severe asthma

In your early 30s, your bones start to lose bone density. Osteoporosis is a condition that is diagnosed when the bones have become so thin that fractures are likely to occur. Women are more at risk than men.

Regular walking can help you maintain and build bone strength, because it is a load-bearing exercise (see page 104). To keep your bones strong you should take part in load-bearing exercise every day. However, if you want to build your bone density, you should increase the amount of load you place on your body over the weeks. This doesn't mean you have to walk faster; you can achieve better results by incorporating hills or some other form of resistance, such as on sand. Try to complement your daily walking with other gentle load-bearing exercises, such as gentle jogging, stair-climbing, dancing, step aerobics, racket sports and jumping rope. The only

## Week 1

Take three short walks this week, lasting about 10 to 15 minutes each. These will be your **Daily Dose**. Concentrate on getting used to the idea of a daily walk.

**Day 1** Go for one 10-minute walk. Choose a flat and even surface and take it at whatever speed feels comfortable.

**Day 2** Walk for 10 minutes today, using the same route you walked on Day 1. This time concentrate on technique and make sure that your posture is good (see page 27)—focus on keeping your abdomen pulled in to keep your back strong.

**Day 3** Go for a 15-minute walk, and choose a different route this time. Keep to a moderate pace and think about your posture (see pages 26 to 27).

If you have been told by your doctor that your bones are thin, use this week to get used to the idea that walking is something that will help you with your condition. Think positively about how the impact of the exercise is strengthening your weight-bearing bones. It's important to remember that it's healthier to walk regularly than to sit at home and let your bones and muscles become weak. If you experience any pain that persists when you stop exercising, contact your doctor.

## Week 2

Walk your **Daily Dose** at a "light-to-moderate" level (RPE of 11 to 13) or at about 55 to 65 percent of your maximum heart rate every day this week, but try to increase three of these walks to 20 minutes.

While you're walking, concentrate on the swing of your arms and remember to walk tall to build up the muscles around your spine. The more supported your spine, the more protected it is against stoops and fractures.

If at any time you're finding it difficult to get out and about, replace your **Daily Dose** with 10 minutes of stair-climbing or a minute of jumping rope.

> **Daily Dose**
> Try to walk for at least 10 minutes a day, building up to 20 minutes a day in later weeks. Incorporate hills into your walks whenever possible.

## HRT: WHAT THE EXPERTS SAY

According to research by the American Society of Bone and Mineral Research, women who exercise regularly and are on Hormone Replacement Therapy (HRT) improve the mineral density in their bones more than women who are only on HRT or exercise. Compared with those who don't exercise, active women cut their risk of fractures in half.

sports to avoid are contact sports or those which have a high risk of a fall. Walking is also a great exercise for improving your balance, which is important if you have thin bones, as every fall has a potential for bone breaks. Supplement your program with the balance exercise on page 179 once a week. If your balance is poor perform the exercise with a friend or stand a chair next to you for support.

## Weeks 3 to 4

Continue with your **Daily Dose**, but increase four of the walks to 20 minutes. Do some of these walks on the same route. This will allow you to concentrate fully on your posture and technique rather than being distracted by unfamiliar surroundings.

Keep to flat and even surfaces so that you're building up your muscles and bones without putting undue pressure on them.

## Weeks 5 to 7

Build up your **Daily Dose** to five 20-minute walks each week. Introduce gentle hills to at least two of these walks. An incline increases the force of gravity you're working against, so therefore the load you're putting on your skeleton. Walking uphill helps you build up the muscles around your hips also, which is important because hips are vulnerable areas for fractures. The pace does not need to be fast, because this level of walking will be improving your musculoskeletal fitness (the strength of your muscles and bones) by the distance you walk, not the intensity of exercise.

## Weeks 8 to 10+

Your **Daily Dose** should now be 20 minutes every day. This can be broken down into two periods of 10 minutes each day.

Introduce a few more hills to your walking program, or tackle some steeper hills. If there are no hills in your area, then increase the amount of stair-climbing. Try also to complement your walking with other load-bearing exercises, such as dancing or jumping rope.

# WALKING AWAY FROM **STRESS**

**Use this program if:**

▶ You have difficulty falling asleep or wake through the night with things on your mind

▶ You regularly suffer from headaches, migraines, neck or back pain or from other conditions that may be induced by stress, such as Irritable Bowel Syndrome (IBS)

▶ You have high blood pressure

▶ You feel overwhelmed or unable to cope with small challenges and fear change

▶ You find that you rely on alcohol or cigarettes to relax you, particularly if you've had a hard day

Do you often feel tired yet continue to rush around, sorting out the details of everyday life? Do you feel overwhelmed by the amount of bills, emails, paperwork and housework you have to deal with? Are you compromising your goals to accommodate others' demands? These are classic causes of stress. This program has been designed to show how regular walking can help reduce the stress in your life.

Anxiety has become a fact of life for many of us, and is a barrier to achieving tranquillity and contentment. Sometimes problems clutter our minds like junk in a messy garage. And like that junk, if not put to good use or thrown away, these problems can build up. A quick solution is to close the door and run away, but this only makes matters worse. The answer is to set aside time every day to be by yourself, think things through, order your thoughts and start to solve

## Week 1

On top of your **Daily Dose**, try to make time in your week for at least two 20-minute walks. By going for a walk on your own terms, for your own benefit, you've cleared the first hurdle—you believe in yourself, are thinking about addressing your own needs and are taking control. It's a statement both to you and to others. So this week, just get out.

## Week 2

At a minimum, walk your **Daily Dose**, building up to 20 minutes, if possible, on two occasions.

In addition, find time to go for a slightly longer walk of at least 30 minutes. As you walk, let your thoughts wander for a while without any specific direction. Then, try to concentrate on the people, buildings or trees you pass. Does your mind take you back to the same thoughts and problems, no matter what your eye is focusing on? If so, then you can be sure that these are the important issues in your life. Write them down and put them into categories, depending on whether they're work-related, money worries or family issues. Start to think about practical solutions for these problems while using this program.

## Weeks 3 to 4

Over these two weeks, continue with your minumum **Daily Dose**.

Aim to add two 45-minute walks each week. Warm up, then step up the pace and walk as quickly as you can for as long as you can manage. This will help you to remove any aggression and pent-up emotion and make you focus on the physical act of walking rather than on your emotional worries.

After the fast burst, slow down and bring your mind back to your problems. If your thought process starts, "I really ought to…" then you're on the wrong track. "Ought" reflects an action based on duty or guilt. Use your walking to rid yourself of these associations.

> **Daily Dose**
> Take a walk for 10 minutes every day to give yourself time to think. Use this time to empty your mind of anything that is troubling you. Try to avoid traffic and busy streets.

problems. In time, this will help you to feel more able to cope with life. If you are suffering from the physical symptoms of stress, such as tense shoulders, headaches and poor sleep, walking can help by promoting relaxation and releasing endorphins, which bring an immediate sense of well-being.

## STEPS TO EASE STRESS

Many anxieties can be reduced simply by managing your life more effectively. Think about these as you walk.

▶ **Step 1** Believe in yourself and convince yourself that you can take control of your life.

▶ **Step 2** Think about all the issues that could be causing your stress, whether they're work-related, money worries, health concerns, family pressures or personal conflicts. Put them into categories.

▶ **Step 3** Take each category and think about practical changes you can make. Start to deal specifically with straightforward problems.

▶ **Step 4** Consider whether outside help, such as a baby-sitter, financial advisor or just the ear of a good friend, could be beneficial to you.

## Weeks 5 to 6

You should be trying to walk whenever you get the chance, particularly if there are still times when things overwhelm you. Increase the duration of your **Daily Dose** to 15 to 20 minutes at least three or four times a week.

If you feel that your workload or other work-related problems are the main causes of your stress, make sure you use your lunch break as a time to go for a walk, not to catch up on all the things you haven't done in the office. Even a 15-minute walk will give you a clearer head and help you to deal more efficiently with your work once you get back to the office.

Go also for one or two longer walks of about 1 hour each week. Use this time to work out how to deal with the problems you've identified. Start with the easiest problem, however trivial. Come back from the walk and make that difficult phone call or write that sensitive letter. Don't put it off any longer. Then move on to some of the more deep-rooted problems. Long walks will help your mind to gradually become less cluttered and more calm. This can give you the confidence to deal with bigger problems. Choose routes that take you through green spaces or by water, both of which can help calm your mind.

## Weeks 7 to 10

Your walks can become shorter, but more frequent—four 30-minute walks a week is ideal. As you give your mind space, you'll not only find it easier to think about how you can manage and organize your life, but will also gain a greater sense of perspective.

As you walk, concentrate on the people you pass—there will be those with greater, and others with lesser problems than yours. If you walk in a natural setting also, you may get a sense that you're part of a larger whole, and this can help you put your troubles in perspective. If you feel your stress levels rising again, find the perfect setting and go back to the longer walks of Weeks 5 to 6.

# WALKING BACK TO **HAPPINESS**

**Use this program if:**

▶ You're suffering from depression and undergoing a course of counseling and/or medication but are looking for natural ways of complementing your treatment

▶ You're recovering from depression and feel ready to "get out there"

▶ You want to meet new people, widen your social circle and enjoy new activities as part of your program of recovery from depression

We all want to be happy, yet happiness can be so hard to find. Exercise has been clinically proven to boost the spirits and bring some relief when we are feeling very down and our lives seem out of control.

Many of us will suffer from stress and anxiety at some point in our lives; some of us also may suffer from a feeling of despair, hopelessness and a lack of interest in life. This feeling is depression, an illness generally thought to be caused by a reduction in certain chemicals (neurotransmitters) in the brain. It can be a debilitating condition, but one that can be treated effectively with medication and/or counseling. The symptoms of depression can also be reduced by physical activity, as exercise releases the body's own natural antidepressants, endorphins, which have been shown to play a key role in determining mood and the body's response to stress.

## Week 1

Get out for your **Daily Dose** as often as possible. Don't worry if you don't manage to go out every day; this is your week for getting used to being out and about again.

Find two occasions when you can go for a leisurely walk in a park or a rural setting. Listen closely to sounds (birdsong, a stream, children playing) and observe the sights around you (clouds, colors, trees). Simply try to enjoy the experience of being outside.

## Week 2

Get out for your **Daily Dose** as many days as possible. Don't worry if you don't manage it one day—just take the program at your pace.

Go for three longer walks of 20 to 30 minutes each, varying your route each time. At the end of the week, decide which of these you would like to be your set route, a route you can travel whenever you need space for thinking.

On at least one of these walks, spend time thinking back to a period in your life when you were happy. Try to identify why you were happy at that time. As you walk, remember to clear your mind of thoughts of "what could have been" or "what might possibly be" and focus on what you have now.

## Weeks 3 to 4

Walk your set route at least once each week. Keeping to the same route can help you monitor changes in how you're feeling, as you associate particular landmarks with thoughts you had at that spot on earlier walks.

If you can, go for one longer walk of around 30 to 45 minutes during each of these weeks. Use one of these walks as a social occasion and walk with a friend, even if he or she only joins you for part of the walk. Use the other walk to think about what determines your quality of life. Try to understand that there will always be changes in your life, some good and some bad.

> ### Daily Dose
> A 10-minute walk can be enough to release endorphins and lift your mood. Concentrate on enjoying the present.

As well as introducing you to the psychological benefits of exercise, this program will provide you with a structured way to think about deep-seated issues in your life. Social interaction can provide reassurance, as well as being a way of putting your problems into perspective, so try to coordinate some of these walks with the activities of friends and family: Encourage a friend to walk with you, or use a walk as an opportunity to visit a relative or neighbor.

## NATURAL MOOD-ENHANCERS

A study carried out at Nottingham Trent University, England, published in the *British Journal of Sports Medicine* in 2001, has shown that physical activity probably boosts people's moods thanks to a naturally occurring amphetamine—a stimulant which improves mood and decreases fatigue—released into the bloodstream. Levels of the compound phenylethylamine are nearly 80 percent higher in people after about 30 minutes on a treadmill. People who are depressed have been found to have low levels of these natural amphetamines leading to the conclusion that regular activity will help keep depression at bay and even leave you on a natural high.

## Weeks 5 to 6

Continue with your **Daily Dose**. Try to get out every day, even if only for 5 to 10 minutes. Use this time to take a break from worries and align yourself in the present.

Go for three longer walks during each of these weeks, staying out for at least 30 to 40 minutes. Once you've warmed up on these walks, introduce an element of very fast walking for 5 to 10 minutes. Then, gradually, slow down and think about your feelings. If any negative emotions have come to the surface during your walk, the best thing you can do is to just let go.

Make at least one of the walks a social occasion. If you're feeling particularly low one day don't think that this is not the day for walking with a friend or visiting family. Meeting and chatting with others might be just what you need to help raise your spirits.

Use another of the walks as an opportunity to observe and appreciate nature. Choose a pleasant natural setting, preferably near water or woodland, and think about the animal and plant life around you as you walk. Listen to your deepest thoughts and try to separate these from the superficial stresses in your life.

## Weeks 7 to 10

Continue with at least three long walks of 45 minutes to 1 hour a week in natural settings. Think about positive and negative energy. Positive energy comes from good times spent with family and friends and from making contact with nature. Negative energy comes from feelings such as guilt and greed. Natural settings may help you to recharge your batteries. Make sure you're not working long hours and never finding time to meet with friends or family. You might want to widen your walking circle by joining a group (see page 62).

## Use this program if:

► You have an extremely busy life and can't see how you can fit a program of regular walking into your hectic schedule

► You're a working mom and are trying to juggle a full-time job with looking after the kids

► You're worried you spend too much time at your desk and need something to force you out of the office to get some fresh air

► You're looking for a form of exercise that you can do without driving to a gym or sports hall

► You want something you can do without buying equipment or special clothes

Lack of time is the reason most often given for not exercising. This program shows you that walking is the one activity you can easily fit into your busy day. A **Daily Dose** of 30 minutes can be divided into manageable chunks and you'll still reap the benefits.

Time is precious. What you choose to do with it is up to you. There's no doubt that some of us have a tendency to overwork, spending every available minute at our desks and taking our work home with us. In recent decades, we've seen a work culture develop that views taking a lunch break or leaving work on time as signs of weakness.

Fortunately, things are changing now and employers are beginning to realize that the most productive employees are not always the ones who stay late at the office and work through their lunch hours. In fact, it's the ones who use their leisure time

## Week 1

**Day 1** Take a look at your daily activities and see which you could eliminate. Which television program would you not mind missing? Which responsibility could be delegated? Build some walking time into your day, even if it's just parking the car farther from the office. Go for a lunchtime walk and take your sandwich to the park.

**Day 2** Free up 30 minutes for a brisk walk. Walk to an activity or errand where normally you would use the car, such as shopping or getting to work, or wake up 30 minutes earlier in the morning.

**Day 3** Look for ways to increase intensity by including hills and maintaining the same pace uphill as you do on a flat route. Walk for at least 30 minutes today.

**Day 4** Pencil in 1 hour during the next three days for a longer walk. Do your **Daily Dose**.

**Day 5** If a longer walk was scheduled for today, then complete the hour you set aside. If the walk becomes impossible, at least do your **Daily Dose**.

**Day 6** Unless you have planned your hour-long walk for today, walk briskly for 20 to 30 minutes at a "hard" level (RPE of 15 to 16), or at about 75 to 80 percent of your maximum heart rate.

**Day 7** If you're walking for longer today, concentrate on mixing periods of fast walking with a moderate-to-brisk pace.

## Week 2

Walk every day this week, even if on some days you can manage only 15 minutes at a brisk pace. Take your walking clothes to work to motivate you to walk at lunchtime.

Try to include one longer walk lasting an hour and which includes a hill. Work at a "moderate-to-hard" level (RPE of 13 to 16), or at about 65 to 80 percent of your maximum heart rate.

> ### Daily dose
> Walk briskly for 20 to 30 minutes on all or most days of the week, split into two periods if necessary.

## ADDING INTENSITY

Your walking program can be adapted to whatever time you can spare. Remember that, on the whole, intensity and duration are interchangeable: increased intensity means working harder for a shorter time yet with the same benefits.

► Use your arms more: You'll recruit more muscle and make your heart work harder.

► Walk uphill whenever you can, maintaining a good pace—even a modest incline of 4 percent can burn 3 to 5 more calories per minute than walking on the flat ground.

► Perfect your fast-walking technique so you can cover more ground in less time.

to advantage and look after their health who will perform most effectively overall. Exercising during your lunch hour will leave you more alert and awake throughout the afternoon. Time invested in improving your health is never wasted. You'll be repaid tenfold as your health improves by the day and you continue to be fit and active in your later years.

Make sure you include warm-up and cool-down periods during your walk; skimping on these may lead to injury.

## Weeks 3 to 5

Continue with your minimum **Daily Dose**. Keep practicing your faster walking technique (see page 45), using your arms as much as possible. Include hills in your walk when you can to add intensity, or add resistance by walking on challenging terrain such as sand or muddy ground. Watch your posture when walking uphill (see page 48).

Take two longer walks of 45 to 60 minutes, with at least 20 minutes at a "hard" level.

## Weeks 6 to 12

By now you should have found that time spent walking is never wasted, but is time well spent. You can use it to think creatively about the different aspects of your life. If you join a walking group, you can use the time to socialize. Start noting your walks in a diary. Experts agree that maximum benefits are gained from walking 45 to 60 minutes, three or four times a week at the "moderate-to-hard" level. Make this your goal.

## Weeks 12+

Your total weekly walking time should now be:

30 minutes 3 to 4 days a week, split into two periods, if necessary.

Two longer walks per week of between 45 and 60 minutes, 20 minutes of which should be at a "moderate-to-hard" level.

Try not to let your walking time be taken over by other things. Walking aids relaxation and helps you to think more clearly, both of which will help you use the rest of your time more efficiently.

# WALKING WITH **CHILDREN**

**Use this program if:**

▶ You're concerned that your children spend most of their leisure time playing computer games or surfing the Net and get little physical exercise

▶ Your children show little interest in the outdoors

▶ You're concerned that your children might be becoming overweight

▶ You're looking for an activity to unite the family and benefit the health of everybody

▶ You want to go walking yourself but can't without the children

As leisure pursuits increasingly revolve around the TV or computer screen and most children are driven to school or extracurricular activities, the risk of obesity in children is on the rise. Even if children play a lot of sports, they are unlikely to get as much physical activity as past generations, and this can have serious consequences on their health. If walking becomes a natural part of their lives, this trend can be reversed, helping them to stay at a healthy weight, strengthen their growing bones and develop coordination. Increased outdoor activity also can help children and preteens get away from stresses and strains in their emotional lives and help them to become happier and more balanced in their outlooks.

Passing on your enthusiasm for walking to your children is not always easy. Use your imagination and try to base the walk around a theme, such as

## Weeks 1 to 2

**Week 1** Try for one fairly slow walk of about 1 hour this week. Start with a walk along a river or around a lake, and pause to feed the ducks. This simple start is usually successful as long as there's enough to do and see.

**Week 2** The next walk can be in the parkland or woods. Keep your children's minds active as you go—encourage them to dig in the ground with sticks, organize a treasure hunt, award points for spotting squirrels or mushrooms, play hide-and-seek, climb trees—anything to keep things moving. A toddler should be able to manage about a mile (1.6 km), older children can walk 2 to 3 miles (3.2 to 4.8 km).

## Week 3

Take Frisbees, balls or kites and head for a large open space. Park at least 1 mile (1.6 km) from the final destination, and make the sports and games the focus of the walk. The excitement of games or kite-flying may distract your children from realizing they're on a walk. To avoid thoughts of tiredness or boredom on the return stretch, keep them busy talking about what a good time they had.

## Week 4

A natural-history walk is both entertaining and educational. Bring an identification book, an old white sheet and two plastic containers. Choose a small tree, lay the sheet underneath it and shake the branches. All sorts of strange insects will fall onto the sheet and crawl to the edge. Let the children catch them and put them in the containers for later identification. Older children can help look up and label butterflies, animals and flowers. If you can tie this in with any subject they might be studying at school, then so much the better.

### Daily Dose

Get your children out walking for at least 20 minutes four or five times a week. This could be their walk to and from school if they normally ride the bus or take the subway.

identifying plants or details of the landscape. If there's opposition be firm but allow children some input by giving them options that still include a walk.

The walks here are "once-a-week" walks, because they need planning. It might be best to take toddlers on a walk during the day, and older children on a different kind of walk after school or on the weekend.

## PACKING FOR THE CHILDREN

Most children will need plenty of encouragement to go on a walk. A little extra load for you will be well worth it, so make sure you pack the following:

- **Drinks** Water, juice or a sports drink
- **Snacks** Take healthy options such as fruit, granola bars or popcorn, for when they say "I'm hungry"
- **A large day pack** To carry jackets and pullovers when they are too hot
- **Hats and gloves** For the colder months
- **Spare clothes** Good for when it turns cold or if you're near water
- **Sunscreen** Even for cool, clear days
- **A plastic bag and some wipes** These always come in handy

## Week 5

There's mounting evidence that the sterile environment in which many children are brought up today is contributing to the rise in asthma and eczema. There's no harm in children getting a bit muddy now and again, and, for them, the muddy walk is the one that's not to be missed. Choose a nearby trail, or drive to an appropriate location if necessary. Walk for at least 2 hours. Although splashing in rain puddles (great for creating piles of laundry) may not be your idea of fun, the smiling mud-spattered faces of your children will more than make up for it.

## Weeks 6 to 7

**Week 6** One way to negotiate a "serious" walk with children is with the "serious" picnic at the end of it. For longer walks, make sure you have a jogging stroller or a child carrier for a very young child, if necessary. This means the walk won't be held up if your toddler becomes tired. Try to walk for about 3 hours, including the picnic time. Older children can use the picnic spot as a base for further exploration or games.

**Week 7** If you have easy access to a beach, then there's really no limit to the type and length of walk you can take. Go collect shells or driftwood, or take a long walk at low tide. Try other places to walk, such as a path around a local lake or a mountain trail.

## Weeks 8 to 10

Try to combine as many different types of walk as you can into the week: a "themed" walk lasting several hours; a short walk in the park with toddlers (try to fit in at least three of these a week); walks to and from school (every day if possible) and perhaps a 30-minute walk with an older child, when you'll have the opportunity to talk about any difficulties at school or anything else your child may have on his or her mind.

# PROGRAMS FOR **GROUPS**

*Devising a walking program for a group is a challenging but very rewarding undertaking. The secret is to design a program that caters to several different abilities while ensuring everyone works at their own level.*

Once you've taken the decision to lead a group and done all the research and background work (see pages 60 to 61), it's time to sit down and plan your walks. Programs are useful because they provide structure, allowing you to increase the speed, duration and intensity of the walks over the weeks and so to keep people interested and building their fitness. However, planning a program for a group is complicated by the fact that you have to cater for people of different abilities. This is when techniques such as grading your routes, using leaders and targeted motivation tactics come into play.

## *Grading your routes*

If you're coordinating a walking group it's a good idea to grade your walks according to difficulty. The grades should encompass speed and distance as well as hills and terrain. (Remember that downhill walking can be just as demanding as walking on the flat ground.) You could class your walks as "C," "B" or "A," according to

## Community spirit

*A walking group brings together people of all ages and backgrounds to share their leisure time.*

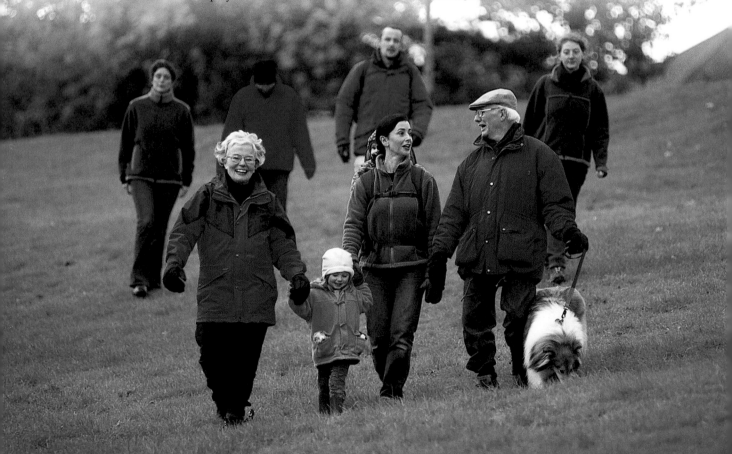

level of difficulty. "C" walks would be entirely on the flat terrain, with no fences and at a pace of no more than 2.5 to 3 mph (4 to 4.8 km/h), "B" walks would be primarily on the flat ground, but with moderate inclines built in, and "A" walks would include several hills and cover rough paths and fields. Alternatively, use grading systems such as "Beginners," "Intermediate" and "Advanced" or "Blue," "Red" and "Black." Make sure you try out your routes before you set them for your group both to assess their difficulty and so that you can provide information such as particular weather or surface conditions.

## Following the leader

If you split a group up to follow different routes you may need more than two leaders. The most important leader is always the one at the back of the group whose job it is to walk at the pace of the slowest, encouraging and motivating them. Walkie-talkies are a great way for leaders to keep in touch with each other throughout the walk and are essential if leaders want to make any changes to the preplanned route—for example, if the group is going faster or slower than anticipated.

## Motivating others

If you're enjoying your walking and are eager to encourage family and friends, put yourself in the position of someone who leads a sedentary lifestyle, in order to understand what will motivate them. There's no point handing out timetables of walks if the people you're targeting have not even thought about taking up walking. A leaflet about the benefits of walking would be better for this group and the timetables reserved for people who have already decided to join you.

A good motivating strategy is to encourage walkers to buddy-up with someone of similar ability. Familiarize walkers with the road-safety guidelines on page 69 and make sure you tell your group before you set off about any dangerous road crossings, uneven footpaths or potholes along the way.

*Walkers' tips*

# ROUTES FOR MIXED-ABILITY GROUPS

### A figure of "8"
*The slower walkers can walk the bottom half of the "8" while the faster walkers walk the full distance.*

### Open spaces
*Parks and fields are ideal for sending the faster walkers around the perimeter and the slower walkers straight across the area.*

### Focal points and markers
*Include several natural landmarks or ones you've placed yourself. Faster walkers reaching these points can walk back and forth between them or turn around and walk to the back of the group.*

### Varied landscapes
*Make faster walkers follow a more challenging route, such as going up and down a hill, to give the slower walkers time to catch up. If you stop for a break, allow the slower walkers time to catch up and have a break before everyone starts off again.*

# PROGRAMS FOR **GROUPS**

Whatever the level of the group you're working with, for the first few weeks of your walking program it's better to underwork rather than overwork them. If people complain that they do not find the walks challenging enough, you can ask those individuals to double-back on certain sections of the walk, particularly hills. If you are working with more than one group, remember that programs for different levels and abilities can be run simultaneously each week. Try to keep all walks to an hour or less so that people can partake several times per week even if they have a busy life.

### Beginner's program

For an inexperienced group concentrate on routes that are on the level. Try to avoid fences and difficult terrain. Start with local routes of about 1 to 2 miles (1.6 to 3.2 km) in length.

### Intermediate program

Choose a route of about 3 to 4 miles (4.8 to 6.4 km) for your intermediate or "B" group. The walkers in this group will be ready to tackle moderate slopes, although you should still make sure that the majority of your walk is on good, even terrain so that they can concentrate on building up their speeds. Teach good form and correct posture before increasing the pace. Use some short bursts of faster walking to get them used to working unfamiliar muscle groups.

### Advanced program

An advanced or "A" walking group is the easiest to manage as most group members will be self-motivated and already walking with regularity and enthusiasm. As well as adding hills to their walks you can cover rougher paths and fields. Choose routes of around 5 to 6 miles (8 to 9.6 km). Many people find that they "hit the wall" at a particular walking pace (see page 155 for advice on getting through this barrier).

## BEGINNER'S PROGRAM

### Week 1

Start off with a short walk on level ground. Aim for a walk that lasts approximately 30 minutes, but try to think in advance of ways of lengthening it or shortening it in case you've underestimated or overestimated the group's capabilities. Concentrate on teaching good technique and posture. Introduce the group to fast walking in a short, five-minute burst, instructing your participants to walk "as if they were late for an appointment." Remember the warm-up and cool-down. Beginners will need a longer warm-up than more advanced walkers.

### Weeks 2 to 10

Continue with fairly short, even routes over these weeks but gradually introduce longer periods of fast walking: increasing from 10 minutes in week 2 to 20 minutes in week 10. During this section the group should be working at a "moderate" level (RPE of 13 to 14), or at about 65 to 70 percent of the estimated maximum heart rate. Use as many different routes as you can, to give the group variety (for ideas, see page 61), but stick to mainly level ground.

### Weeks 10+

Increase the distance you cover and increase the durations of your walks from 30 minutes to 45 minutes. Include at least 20 to 25 minutes at a brisk pace. RPE should be between 13 and 16, or about 65 to 80 percent of the estimated maximum heart rate.

# **INTERMEDIATE** PROGRAM

## Week 1

Intermediate-level walks should last between 45 and 60 minutes. The time/intensity principle still applies—walking faster for a shorter period will bring the same benefits as walking more slowly for a longer period. Routes that form a figure of "8" are particularly good for an intermediate group, as this is the category most likely to become spread out. Look for other ways of regrouping, using techniques such as routes that allow people to walk back and forth between two close markers. Managing your group in this way will give those at the back of the group the chance to catch up or get ahead.

## Weeks 2 to10

Introduce a fast section to your walks, working at a "hard" level (RPE of 15 to 16) or at about 75 to 80 percent of maximum heart rate, and gradually increase the duration of this section from 15 to 20 minutes in the early weeks to 20 to 30 minutes by week 10. Add intensity by varying the terrain and including hills. Concentrate on teaching good form, particularly when climbing hills (see page 48).

## Weeks 10+

Your walkers are now ready to move on to more demanding walks, either with steeper hills or at a faster pace. Look for fun ways to increase their speeds (all the while maintaining good form) by introducing races over short distances. This could take the form of a time trial over 1 mile (1.6 km) at a pace that is fast but does not overexert them.

# **ADVANCED** PROGRAM

## Week 1

Check your walkers' forms. Even though they may be regular walkers, this does not mean that they have good walking techniques. Remind them of the need to warm up and cool down. Make sure that the whole group walks at a "moderate" level for the first 5 to 8 minutes of the walk. Even good walkers take different amounts of time to warm up. It's at the beginning of the walk that the greatest differences in ability manifest themselves. If some walkers do set off at a very fast pace, ask them to double-back after 5 minutes to give the rest of the group time to catch up.

## Weeks 2 to 10

An "A" group often will contain competitive participants. You need to seek out those who are not and make sure that they do not feel inadequate, while at the same time exploiting the enthusiasm of the others. Build in 10-to-20 minute stretches of very fast walking, but remind all participants that the only people they are competing against are themselves. Red faces are usually a sign of healthy exertion rather than overexertion. Look out for people who go pale or whose breathing is labored.

## Weeks 10+

Keep monitoring the level of the group as a whole. Make sure the majority of your walks are ones that everyone is happy with, but build in at least one long walk, which includes a 10-minute fast walk uphill, to stretch them.

# ADDITIONAL FITNESS TESTS

*Tests of your cardiovascular fitness and weight are useful preparations for your program (see pages 140 to 147), but you can also measure improvements in your flexibility, balance and strength using these tests.*

As with the measured-track and weight tests introduced earlier in the chapter, you'll get the most out of these tests if you try them before you begin your program, and then retest yourself at regular intervals. Use the grids on pages 182 to 183 to record your progress. The other advantage of incorporating these tests in your weekly or monthly program is that they are exercises in themselves, which will help to improve your fitness in these areas.

## How flexible are you?

The range of movement you have in your tendons and muscles determines how easily you can perform everyday tasks, including walking. Our flexibility declines as we get older, but the good news is that it can be reversed through regular stretching. Greater flexibility in your legs also leads to an improved walking technique, allowing you to increase your stride length and frequency and, consequently, get more from

## Reach test

*This is an approximate gauge of the flexibility in your lower back and hamstring muscles at the backs of your thighs—muscles and tendons that help to determine your stride length and posture. If you have a bad back or pain in these areas, do not do this test. If you experience any pain during the stretch, stop immediately.*

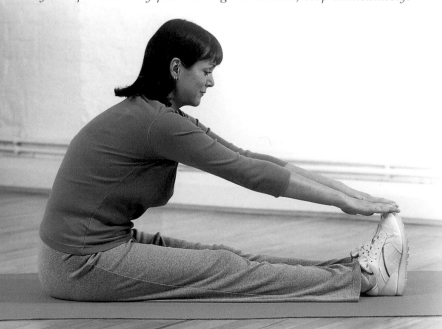

Sit on the floor and stretch your legs out in front of you. Keeping the toes pointing up and your legs straight and together, reach forward to touch your toes. It may feel uncomfortable but should not be painful.

▶ If you can't reach your toes, you have below-average lower-back and hamstring flexibility.

▶ If you can reach your toes but it's uncomfortable, you have average lower-back and hamstring flexibility.

▶ If you can reach your toes without discomfort, you have above-average lower-back and hamstring flexibility.

your walks (see page 33). Stretching will occur naturally when you walk, but also when you perform your cool-down routine (see pages 40 to 43), so test your flexibility regularly to see how much you're benefiting from your walks.

## How good is your balance?

As people get older, they often find that their sense of balance deteriorates, leading to an increased risk of falls and injuries. Consequently, balance is an important element of total fitness. It's affected by many things, but particularly strength, flexibility and the function of special cells throughout the body, called proprioceptors. These are sense cells located in the sensory nerve endings within the muscles, tendons and joints, and also in the hair cells of the balance organ of the inner ear. They detect changes in muscle tension and movement and continually relay this information to the spinal cord and brain. The brain then makes any necessary adjustments in muscle contraction to make sure posture and balance are maintained.

As with many parts of your body, these balance cells become less sensitive the less they are used. Luckily, walking requires you to use these cells, so it's an excellent way of restoring and maintaining good balance and posture. Repeating the test below will also bring improvements and will be a particularly useful addition to your walking routine if you suffer from osteoporosis (see page 105).

## Balance test

*Ask someone to help you with this test. If you feel that your balance is particularly poor, ask the person to stand behind you with his or her arms outstretched to catch you if you look like you're going to fall.*

Stand up straight with your arms by your side. While the other person times you, lift one leg and rest the sole of your foot against your standing leg, just below the knee. Now close your eyes, and see how long you can stay on one leg. Try this three times and record your best time. Perform this test regularly to improve your balance.

▶ If you managed less than 2 seconds, your balance is below average.
▶ If you managed between 2 and 5 seconds, your balance is average.
▶ If you managed more than 5 seconds, your balance is above average.

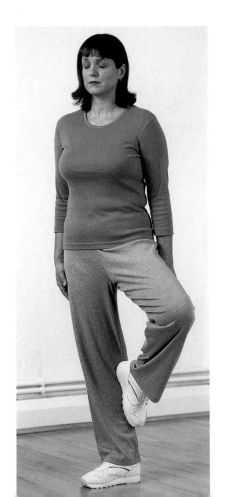

## How strong are you?

Fitness professionals consider two aspects when talking about "strength": one is muscular strength and the other is muscular endurance. "Muscular strength" refers to the amount of force your muscles can exert in one try; it would test, for example, the heaviest weight you could lift. "Muscular endurance," on the other hand, refers to your muscles' ability to keep working over time, so it tests how often or for how long you can repeat an activity. Endurance is what is necessary when walking—maintaining your posture or moving your body weight up a hill, for example.

This section gives you two strength tests: The wall-sit test examines the muscles of your lower body; the push-up test is a test of the muscles of your upper body. As you increase your level of walking you will build the strength and endurance of your lower body.

Repeat the wall-sit test after three months of walking and you should see an improvement. To build your upper-body strength and endurance, concentrate on pumping your arms, use poles as you walk or add some push-ups or wall-presses into your cool-down (see box, opposite). Building your muscles in this way will make you look more toned and will raise your basal metabolic rate (see page 159), which, in turn, will help with weight loss.

Muscular endurance tests should be performed only if you're free from illness or injury. If you have high blood pressure, you should consult your physician before attempting any strength work. If you experience any discomfort whatsoever while performing these tests, leave them out or try them with the help of a fitness expert. You can try both tests, or leave out one that you find uncomfortable.

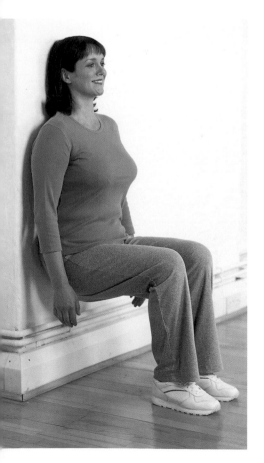

## Wall-sit test

*This is a great way to see how strong your thighs are. You'll need a stopwatch or watch and a wall to lean against. However, if you suffer from knee problems or high blood pressure, avoid this test.*

Stand with your feet about 2 ft (0.6 m) away from a wall. Lean your back flat against the wall. Keeping your back straight, gradually bend your knees and slide your back down the wall until your knees are bent at about 90 degrees, as if you were sitting on a chair. Time how long you can stay in this position.

► If you can't hold the position for more than 30 seconds, then you have below-average lower-body strength.

► If you can hold the position for 30 to 60 seconds, then you have average lower-body strength.

► If you can hold the position for more than 60 seconds, then you have above-average lower-body strength.

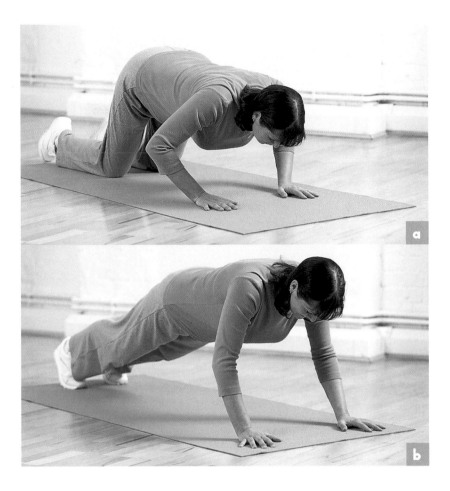

## Push-up test

*There are two versions of this test: Most women and men who are not used to exercise should start with the box push-up; most men and women who are very fit can try the full version.*

**a** *For the box push-up* Get on your hands and knees, with your knees and feet hip-width apart and your hands beneath your shoulders. Your fingers should point forward. Pulling your stomach in and keeping your back straight, use your arms to lower your body. Pause briefly and then push yourself up again, without locking the elbows out straight. See how many push-ups you can perform.

**b** *For the full push-up* Get into a push-up position with your hands beneath your shoulders, and your arms straight, but not locked at the elbows. Your legs should be straight. Keeping your stomach pulled in and your back straight, raise and lower your body using your arms. See how many push-ups you can perform.

▶ If you did fewer than 10 push-ups, you have below-average upper-body strength.
▶ If you managed 10 to 20 push-ups, you have average upper-body strength.
▶ If you managed more than 20 push-ups, you have above-average upper-body strength.

## WALL-PRESSES

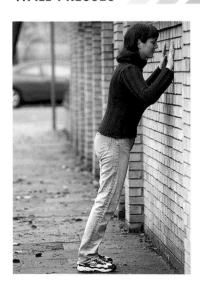

To tone your arms, do ten of these push-ups in each cool-down routine. Stand facing a wall or fence, with your feet hip-width apart. You should be just close enough to place your hands on the wall with your hands shoulder-width apart and your elbows slightly bent. Keeping your back straight, lower your face toward the wall. Pause briefly, then straighten up. Do not lock out your elbows.

# TRACKING YOUR PROGRESS

*Writing things down is an excellent way of keeping yourself motivated. Use the diary and chart on these pages to keep a record of your daily achievements and long-term progress.*

These pages are provided to suggest ways that you can record your progress. If you like to tick things off day by day, then photocopy the Walking Diary as many times as there are weeks in your program. You don't have to fill in all the Time, Distance or Intensity columns, you could just measure the one that you choose to vary (for ways of measuring intensity, see pages 143 to 145). There is space to write in your

weekly goals, which should be steps on the road to your long-term goal (see pages 138 to 139).

The Personal Health Checker is more useful for measuring your long-term progress, but again whatever measure you choose to monitor, it needs to fit your personal goal—if this goal is to be able to walk a certain distance, then recording changes in your weight isn't relevant.

## PERSONAL HEALTH CHECKER

| Date | Resting heart rate (bpm) | Measured-track test: time | Measured-track test: heart rate | Weight (lbs) | Body mass index (BMI rating) |
|---|---|---|---|---|---|
| Starting point | | | | | |
| Week 1 | | | | | |
| Week 2 | | | | | |
| Week 3 | | | | | |
| Week 4 | | | | | |
| Week 5 | | | | | |
| Week 6 | | | | | |
| Week 7 | | | | | |
| Week 8 | | | | | |
| Week 9 | | | | | |
| Week 10 | | | | | |
| Week 11 | | | | | |
| Week 12 | | | | | |
| Month 6 | | | | | |
| Month 9 | | | | | |
| Month 12 | | | | | |

## WALKING DIARY

**Week number**

**Weekly goal**

| Day | Time | Distance | Intensity | Comments |
|-----|------|----------|-----------|----------|
| Monday | | | | |
| Tuesday | | | | |
| Wednesday | | | | |
| Thursday | | | | |
| Friday | | | | |
| Saturday | | | | |
| Sunday | | | | |
| Total | | | | |

**Goal attained?**

**Reward**

| Waist-to-hip ratio | Flexibility (rating) | Lower-body strength (number of sit-ups) | Upper-body strength (number of push-ups) | Balance (number of seconds) |
|---|---|---|---|---|
| | | | | |
| | | | | |
| | | | | |
| | | | | |
| | | | | |
| | | | | |
| | | | | |
| | | | | |
| | | | | |
| | | | | |
| | | | | |
| | | | | |
| | | | | |

# RESOURCES

## APPAREL

### Clothing

*Adidas*
P.O. Box 4015
Beaverton, OR 97076
(503) 972-2300
www.adidas.com

*ASICS TIGER Corporation*
16275 Laguna Canyon Road
Irvine, CA 92618
(800) 678-9435
www.asicscorp.com

*Campmor*
28 Parkway
Box 700
Upper Saddle River, NJ
07458
(201) 825-8300
www.campmor.com

*L.L. Bean Inc.*
Freeport, ME 04033-001
(800) 441-5713
www.llbean.com

*Lands' End*
Lands' End Lane
Dodgeville, WI 53595
(800) 963-4816
www.landsend.com

*Nike*
One Bowerman Drive
Beaverton, OR 97005
(800) 806-6453
www.nike.com

*The North Face*
2013 Farallon Drive
San Leandro, CA 94577
(510) 618-3500
www.thenorthface.com

*Orvis*
1711 Blue Hills Drive
Roanoke, VA 24012
(800) 635-7635
www.orvis.com

*Reebok*
1895 J.W. Foster Boulevard
Canton, MA 02021
(781) 401-5000
www.reebok.com

*REI*
Sumner, WA 98352-0001
(800) 426-4840
www.rei.com

### Fabrics

*DuPont Corporate
Information Center*
Barley Mill Plaza P10
Wilmington, DE 19880-0010
(800) 441-7515

www.dupont.com
*For information on fabrics such
as CoolMax, Cordura, Lycra
and Teflon*

### Footwear

*Merrell Footwear*
9341 Courtland Drive
Rockford, MI 49351
(888) 637-7001
www.merrellboot.com

*Rockport*
1895 J.W. Foster Boulevard
Canton, MA 02021
(800) 762-5767
www.rockport.com

*Teva Sports Sandals*
P.O. Box 968
Flagstaff, AZ 86002
(800) 367-8382
www.tevasandals.com

### Sports Bras

*Champion*
5 New England Drive
Essex, VT 05452
(888) 301-5151
www.championforwomen.
com

## EQUIPMENT

### Backpacks

*Mountainsmith*
18301 W. Colfax Avenue
Building P
Golden, CO 80401
(303) 279-5930
www.mountainsmith.com

*ROKK*
1224 Fern Ridge Parkway
St. Louis, MO 63141
(877) 765-ROKK
www.rokkgear.com

### Bottles, Hydration Systems and Water Purifiers

*CamelBak Products*
1310 Redwood Way
Suite 200
Petaluma, CA 94954
(800) 767-8725
www.camelbak.com

*McNett Corporation*
1411 Meador Avenue
Bellingham, WA 98226
(360) 671-2227
www.mcnett.com

**PUR**
9300 N. 75th Avenue
Minneapolis, MN 55428
(800) 787-5463
www.purwater.com

## Heart-Rate Monitors and Pedometers

*Polar Electro*
370 Crossways Park Drive
Woodbury, NY 11797-2050
(800) 227-1314
www.polarusa.com

*Walk4Life*
11939 Spaulding School
Drive, Unit 1
Plainfield, IL 60544
(888) 422-1806
www.walk4life.com

## Walking Poles and Canes

*Exerstrider Products*
518 Tasman Street, Suite A
Madison, WI 53714-3100
(608) 223-9321
www.exerstrider.com

*Garmont USA*
170 Boyer Circle
Williston, VT 05495
(802) 658-8322
www.garmontusa.com

*Leki USA*
356 Sonwil Drive
Buffalo, NY 14225
(716) 683-1022
www.leki.com

# ORGANIZATIONS

## General

*American Council on Exercise (ACE)*
4851 Paramount Drive
Suite 102
San Diego, CA 92123
(858) 279-8227
(800) 825-3636
www.acefitness.org

*American Volkssport Association*
1001 Pat Booker Road
Suite 101
Universal City, TX 78148
(800) 380-WALK
www.ava.org

*America Walks*
P.O. Box 29103
Portland, OR 97296-9103
(503) 222-1077
www.americawalks.org

*March of Dimes Birth Defects Foundation*
1275 Mamaroneck Avenue
White Plains, NY 10605
(888) 663-4637
www.modimes.org

*The National Academy of Sports Medicine*
Continuing Education
Department
26632 Agoura Road
Calabassas, CA 91302
(818) 878-9203
(866) 292-NASM
www.nasm.org

*National Strength & Conditioning Association*
1955 N. Union Boulevard
Colorado Springs, CO 80909
(719) 632-6722
(800) 815-6826
www.nsca-lift.org

*Partnership for a Walkable America*
National Safety Council
1121 Spring Lake Drive
Itasca, IL 60143-3201
(630) 285-1121
www.nsc.org

*The President's Council on Physical Fitness and Sports*
Department W
200 Independence Avenue
SW, Room 738-H
Washington, DC 20201-0004
(202) 690-9000
www.fitness.gov

## Trails and Parks Organizations

*American Discovery Trail*
P.O. Box 20155
Washington, DC 20041-2155
(800) 663-2387
www.discoverytrail.org

*Appalachian Mountain Club*
5 Joy Street
Boston, MA 02108
www.outdoors.org

*Backroads*
801 Cedar Street
Berkeley, CA 94710-1800
(800) 462-2848
www.backroads.com

*National Coast Trail Association*
5124 N.E. 34th Avenue
Portland, OR 97211
(503) 335-3876
www.coasttrails.org

*National Park Service*
1849 C Street NW
Washington, DC 20240
(202) 208-6843
www.nps.gov

*Parks Canada National Office*
25 Eddy Street
Hull, Quebec
K1A 0M5
(888) 773-8888

www.parkscanada.pch.gc.c
a/parks/main_e.htm
Email:parks_webmasterpch
.gc.ca

*Rails-to-Trails Conservancy*
1100 17th Street NW,
10th Floor
Washington, DC 20036
(202) 331-9696
**www.railtrails.org**

*Trans Canada Trail
Foundation*
43 Westminster Ave. North
Montreal, Quebec
H4X 1Y8
(800) 465-3636
(514) 485-4541
**www.tctrail.ca/trail.htm**
E-mail: info@tctrail.ca

*U.S. Department of
Agriculture Forest Service*
P.O. Box 96090
Washington, DC  20090-
6090
(202) 205-1661
**www.fs.fed.us**

*Volunteer Trailwork
Coalition*
National Trails Day
**www.trailwork.org**

# HEALTH

## General

*Health Canada*
A.L. 0900C2
Ottawa
K1A 0K9
(613) 957-2991
info@hc-sc.gc.ca/

*U.S. Department of Health
and Human Services*
200 Independence Ave. SW
Washington, DC 20201
(202) 619-0257
**www.hhs.gov**

*National Center for Health
Statistics*
Division of Data Services
Hyattsville, MD 20782-2003
(301) 458-4636
**www.cdc.gov/nchs/**

## Arthritis and Osteoporosis

*National Osteoporosis
Foundation*
1232 22nd Street NW
Washington, DC 20037-1292
(202) 223-2226
**www.nof.org**

*Arthritis Foundation*
P.O. Box 7669
Atlanta, GA 30357-0669
(800) 283-7800
**www.arthritis.org**

*Canadian Arthritis
Network*
250 Dundas Street West,
Suite 402
Toronto, Ontario
M5G 1X5
(416) 586-4770
(416) 586-8395
can@mtsinai.on.ca

## Asthma

*Asthma and Allergy
Foundation of America
(AAFA)*
1233 20th Street NW
Suite 402
Washington, DC 20036
(202) 466-7643
**www.aafa.org**

## Back Pain

*American Back Society*
St. Joseph's Professional
Center
2647 International
Boulevard, Suite 401
Oakland, CA 94601
(510) 536-9929
**www.americanbacksoc.org**

*The Back Institute*
1125 South Beverley
Drive 603
Los Angeles, CA 90035
(800) 956-6724
**www.backinstitute.com**

**www.americanspine.com**

## Diabetes

*American Diabetes
Association*
1701 North Beauregard St
Alexandria, VA 22311
(800) 342-2383
**www.diabetes.org**

*Canadian Diabetes
Association*
National Office
15 Toronto Street, Suite 800
Toronto, Ontario, M5C 2E3
(416) 363-3373
(800) 226-8464
info@diabetes.ca

## Foot Health

*FootSmart*
P.O. Box 922908
Norcross, GA 30010-2908
(800) 870-7149
**www.footsmart.com**

## Heart Health

*American Heart Association*
National Center
7272 Greenville Avenue
Dallas, TX 75231
(800) AHA-USA1
**www.americanheart.org**

*Heart and Stroke
Foundation of Canada*
222 Queen Street, Suite 1402
Ottawa, ON K1P 5V9
(613) 569-4361
**www.heartandstroke.ca/**

## OTHER RESOURCES

### Advanced Walking

*Road Runner Sports*
Customer Service
5549 Copley Drive
San Diego, CA 92111
(858) 636-7650
www.roadrunnersports.com

### Hiking, Backpacking and Orienteering

*American Hiking Society*
1422 Fenwick Lane
Silver Spring, MD 29010
(301) 565-6704
www.americanhiking.org

*U.S. Orienteering Federation*
P.O. Box 1444
Forest Park, GA 30298-1444
(404) 363-2110
www.us.orienteering.org

### Mall Walking

*The National Organization of Mall Walkers*
P.O. Box 191
Hermann, MO 65041
(573) 486-3945

*WalkSport America*
P.O. Box 16325
St. Paul, MN 55116
(800) 757-WALK (9255)
www.walksport.com

## Maps

*DeLorme Mapping*
(800) 452-5931
*Supplier of state road atlases*

*Map Express*
P.O. Box 280445
Lakewood, CO 80228
(800) 627-0039
www.mapexp.com

*Raven Maps*
(800) 237-0798
www.ravenmaps.com

*A World of Maps Inc.*
6820 N. Florida Avenue
Tampa, FL 33604
(800) 226-2771
www.aworldofmaps.com

*U.S. Geological Survey*
Information Services
Box 25286, Denver Federal Center
Denver, CO 80225
(800) 435-7627
www.usgs.gov

## Publications

*Backpacker Magazine*
Rodale Inc.
33 E. Minor Street
Emmaus, PA 19098
(610) 967-5171
www.backpacker.com

*EXPLORE magazine*
c/o INDAS
P.O. Box 737
Markham, Ontario
L3P 8A6
(800) 946-0406
www.explore.mag.com

*Fitness Magazine*
375 Lexington Avenue
New York, NY 10017-5514
www.fitnessmagazine.com

*Outside magazine*
400 Market Street
Santa Fe, NM 87501
(505) 989-7100
www.outsidemag.com/magazine/

## Walking Tapes

*Sports Music*
P.O. Box 769689
Roswell, GA 30076
(800) 878-4764
www.sportsmusic.com

*ToneUp Music*
P.O. Box 62025
Santa Barbara, CA 93160-2025
www.walktunes.com

*WalkMate*
P.O. Box 241
Whitby, Ontario
L1N 5S1
www.walkmate.ca

## Walking Vacations

*Specialty Travel Index*
305 San Anselmo Avenue
Suite 313
San Anselmo, CA 94960
(415) 459-4900
www.specialtytravel.com

*The Wayfarers*
172 Bellevue Avenue
Newport, RI 02840
(800) 249-4620
www.walkingvacations.com

## Helpful Websites

www.cardiosport.com
www.gorp.com
www.heeltotoe.com
www.racewalk.com
www.teamoregon.com
www.trailwalk.com
www.thewalkingsite.com
www.walking.about.com
www.walkingstuff.com
www.yahoo.com/recreation/outdoors/walking
www.a1trails.com/hiking/hike_can.html

# INDEX

# ACKNOWLEDGMENTS

**Carroll & Brown would like to thank:**

Additional design and editorial
assistance *Emily Cook, Roland Codd
and Fiona Screen*
Production Manager *Karol Davies*
Production Controller *Nigel Reed*
Computer Management *Paul Stradling*
Picture Researcher *Sandra Schneider*
Indexer *Sue Bosanko*


Photographic props
*Nickson's Countrywear Ltd.
16 Church Street, Caversham
Reading, Berkshire RG4 8AU
www.country-catalogue.co.uk
Tel: 0118 9463804*


Models *Steven Bailey, Sarah Cooke,
Mark Curnock, Martin Humphreys,
Anne Jabre, Sophie Kelly, Linda Noble,
Jeseama Owen, Knole Pirt, Lesley Pirt
and Megan Selmes*


Hair and make-up *Jeseama Owen*

**Picture credits**

Front cover Getty Images
Back cover (bottom)hf holidays

P5 (right) hf holidays
P8 (left) hf holidays
P9 hf holidays
P10 Getty Images
P11 (left) hf holidays, (right) Getty
    Images
P12 (left) Getty Images
p15 (top) hf holidays
P17 Eye of Science/SPL
P25 Getty Images
P26 provided by Montrail,Inc.USA
P28 (left) Getty Images, (right)Getty
    Images
P29 Getty Images
P30 Trail Magazine Tom Bailey
P35 Manfred Kage/SPL
P46/7 Tourism New Zealand
P47 Telegraph Colour Library
P51 courtesy of ATG Oxford
P56 (right) The Countryside
    Agency/Grant Pritchard
P60 The Countryside Agency/Grant
    Pritchard
P62 The Countryside Agency/Grant
    Pritchard
P63 Gilda Pacitti
P64 (top) hf holidays, (left)courtesy of

ATG Oxford, (bottom) Gilda Pacitti
P64/5 courtesy of ATG Oxford
P67 (top) Axiom/ Joe Beynon,
    (bottom)courtesy of ATG Oxford
P69 The Countryside Agency/Grant
    Pritchard
P70 Walk Sport America out of
    St.Paul,Minnesota
P75 Viekka Gustafsson
P76 courtesy of ATG Oxford
P80 Tourism New Zealand
P81 Trail Magazine/Tom Bailey
P82 (left,right)Trail Magazine/Tom
    Bailey
P86 The Countryside Agency/Grant
    Pritchard
P87 Rex Features
P90 John Walsh/SPL
P98 (top)Philippe Plailly/Eurelios/SPL
P102 Damien Lovegrove/SPL
P104 Prof.P.Motta/Deptof
    Anatomy/University 'La
    Sapienza', Rome/SPL
P116 Mauro Fermariello/SPL
P129 Dr Jeremy Burgess/SPL
P135 hf holidays
P143 hf holidays
P144 courtesy of Polar heart rate
    monitors
P 159 Dr Alfred Pasieka/SPL

All other photographs by Jules Selmes